Making Sense of Fibromyalgia

Making Sense of Fibromyalgia

Second Edition

DANIEL J. WALLACE, MD

Associate Director, Rheumatology Fellowship Program

Clinical Professor of Medicine

Cedars-Sinai Medical Center

David Geffen School of Medicine at UCLA

Los Angeles, California

JANICE BROCK WALLACE, MPA

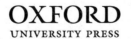
OXFORD

UNIVERSITY PRESS

OXFORD

UNIVERSITY PRESS

Oxford University Press is a department of the University of Oxford.
It furthers the University's objective of excellence in research, scholarship,
and education by publishing worldwide.

Oxford   New York

Auckland   Cape Town   Dar es Salaam   Hong Kong   Karachi
Kuala Lumpur   Madrid   Melbourne   Mexico City   Nairobi
New Delhi   Shanghai   Taipei   Toronto

With offices in

Argentina   Austria   Brazil   Chile   Czech Republic   France   Greece
Guatemala   Hungary   Italy   Japan   Poland   Portugal   Singapore
South Korea   Switzerland   Thailand   Turkey   Ukraine   Vietnam

Oxford is a registered trademark of Oxford University Press
in the UK and certain other countries.

Published in the United States of America by
Oxford University Press
198 Madison Avenue, New York, NY 10016

© Oxford University Press 1999, 2014

Library of Congress Cataloging-in-Publication Data
Wallace, Daniel J. (Daniel Jeffrey), 1949–
Making sense of fibromyalgia / Daniel J. Wallace, MD, associate director, Rheumatology Fellowship
Program, clinical professor of medicine, Cedars-Sinai Medical Center, David Geffen School of
Medicine at UCLA, Los Angeles, California, Janice Brock Wallace, MPA.—Second edition.
pages cm
Includes bibliographical references and index.
ISBN 978–0–19–932176–6
1. Fibromyalgia—Popular works.   I. Wallace, Janice Brock.   II. Title.
RC927.3.W34 2014
616.7'42—dc23
2013024784

1 3 5 7 9 8 6 4 2
Printed in the United States of America
on acid-free paper

Contents

Foreword

Making Sense of Fibromyalgia is a well-written compendium directed to the millions with severe fatigue, muscular pain, poor sleep patterns, and the other symptoms characteristic of fibromyalgia. While there is continuing debate in the medical and research community about the causes and treatments for this misunderstood syndrome, Dr. Daniel J. Wallace's clinical experience and studied review of the current literature have enabled him to produce a book that discusses many of the current theories and understandings.

Dr. Wallace's specific discussions on the diagnostic elements; procedures that support, differentiate, and exclude fibromyalgia as a primary or secondary condition; and specific therapies and their expected efficacies continue the learning process for the reader and provide hope through better understanding of this often maligned condition.

This is an important book that provides a nice complement to the Arthritis Foundation's own publication *Your Personal Guide to Living with Fibromyalgia.* The Arthritis Foundation, Southern California Chapter, is grateful to Dr. Daniel J. Wallace and Oxford University Press for their support of our program for people with fibromyalgia through donations from the sale of this book, *Making Sense of Fibromyalgia.*

Medical & Scientific Committee
Arthritis Foundation, Southern California Chapter
Los Angeles, California

Preface to the Second Edition

To talk of diseases is a sort of Arabian Night's entertainment
Sir William Osler (1849–1919)

Among the childhood pastimes we enjoyed was a peculiar board game known as "Uncle Wiggily" (Fig. 1). Its premise seems quaint when viewed from an adult perspective many years later, but the first player enabling Uncle Wiggily to reach Doc Possum's house so that his rheumatism could be treated was the winner. Along the way, all sorts of nostrums, barriers, diversions, and misinformation deterred Uncle Wiggily from his goal. What, we asked our child's mind, was *rheumatism?* This mysterious, all-encompassing term could apply to fibromyalgia. Fibromyalgia is a syndrome that defies our usual concepts of a disorder and is classified by the Arthritis Foundation as a form of "soft tissue rheumatism." The purpose of this monograph is to enable you to help yourself; to make it easier to work with your doctor and other allied health professionals; to improve the way you feel; and to promote a better quality of life. To begin, there are several reasons why fibromyalgia is plagued by misunderstanding:

- Although it is now recognized as a legitimate syndrome by the American Medical Association, the American College of Rheumatology, the Arthritis Foundation, and the American College of Physicians, as well as the World Health Organization, some doctors still question its existence. This is largely a consequence of incomplete medical training that was (and often still is) primarily hospital-based. Outpatient (office-based) clinical medicine training, which included fibromyalgia, was largely overlooked. Patients are rarely, if ever, hospitalized for fibromyalgia. Also, statistically validated criteria for defining fibromyalgia were not endorsed by organized medicine until 1990.
- Fibromyalgia patients often have normal blood tests and imaging studies and are thought by some health care professionals to make up many of their symptoms. Certain doctors consider fibromyalgia patients to be

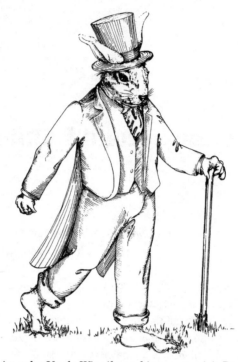

Fig. 1. *An achy Uncle Wiggily on his way to visit Doc Possum.*

hypochondriacs or seekers of medical attention for purposes of litigation or secondary gain. Fortunately, there are now reproducible tests documenting that these complaints are real and studies showing that hypochondriasis is extremely rare in fibromyalgia.

- Six million people in the United States meet the criteria for fibromyalgia. On average, they saw about four doctors before they were correctly diagnosed, and many were convinced they had a life-threatening illness such as a body-wide cancer. Fibromyalgia is a combination of pain, fatigue, and systemic symptoms. Ten million patient visits to doctors every year in the United States are for pain; $600 billion is spent annually to diagnose or manage chronic pain, including litigation fees. One group has estimated that patients with fibromyalgia run up $20 billion in medical expenses annually. Some 10% of US adults have moderate pain and 1% have severe pain; 12% have functional disability due to chronic pain. Additionally, at any visit, 15% of all patients tell their doctor they are tired. There is a paucity of reliable, detailed information about the fibromyalgia syndrome that patients can use to help themselves or others.

- Many employers do not realize that fibromyalgia is a treatable workplace problem. It can impair job performance even though its symptoms and signs are invisible. Over a billion workdays costing $300 billion are lost annually due to pain and 50 million Americans are partially disabled due to chronic pain. Up to 10% of fibromyalgia patients are totally disabled, 30% require job modifications, and 30% have to change their job in order to remain employed. Appropriate treatment, workstation modifications, and counseling could save the American public hundreds of millions of dollars, improve our productivity, and maintain the self-esteem of the fibromyalgia sufferer.

- Every year, over $13 billion is spent out of pocket for non-insurance-reimbursed care by alternative medicine physicians and other caregivers in the United States. Some of this is spent by fibromyalgia patients who are frustrated by the lack of attention, knowledge, and concern of their primary care and specialist physicians.

- In our opinion, there is a relative shortage of rheumatologists, the subspecialists within internal medicine who deal with fibromyalgia, and too little research is ongoing to understand its cause, diagnosis, and treatment. In 2011, the National Institutes of Health allocated only $12 million for fibromyalgia research.

This book is intended not only for fibromyalgia patients, but also for their loved ones, primary care physicians, allied health professionals (nurses, social workers, dentists, physical therapists, psychologists, occupational therapists, vocational rehabilitation counselors, physician assistants, chiropractors, and dietitians), and other people who care about them. A few portions of this book were originally published in a monograph I wrote with Dan Clauw for the Oxford American Rheumatology Library in 2009. Some of Dr Clauw's insights are included verbatim in this update.

Since the original iteration of this concept, originally published as *Making Sense of Fibromyalgia,* was written 15 years ago, many advances have been made in fibromyalogy. This includes three FDA approved medications and over 10,000 peer-reviewed publications. We hope that you find this update informative and useful.

Los Angeles, California
September, 2013

Fibromyalgia Made Simple

A Parable

Pain has an element of blank;
It cannot recollect
When it began, or if there were
A day when it was not.
It has no future but itself
Its infinite realms contain
Its past, enlightened to perceive
New periods of pain.

Emily Dickinson (1830–1886)
Pain Has an Element of Blank

If you have the chronic pain of fibromyalgia, you may be frustrated by the lack of understanding shown by people around you. This is particularly true of the people you live and work with. If only they could feel for one day how you feel all year! Pain has no memory and no mercy. Is it like a bad flu or a severe headache? How can you find the words to describe it? You might wish to recite this short explanation; the next 200 pages provide the details.

Picture your body as being a series of electrical circuits. Suppose that you have the unfortunate tendency to injure your shoulder repeatedly. What happens? As part of a chronic pain response, a wire goes from the shoulder to your spine, and a second wire then travels up the spinal cord to your brain. The brain receives a signal that says, "I hurt my shoulder; let me do something about it." The brain then makes a chemical or chemicals that suppress the pain. It wires a signal back down the spinal column, and a second wire returns to the shoulder. The chemical is released, and the pain gets better or goes away.

What happens in fibromyalgia? Your body becomes "cross-circuited" (Fig. 2). The body gets flooded with "input" circuits giving it information. The spinal cord can't sort out and filter these signals. Larger circuits close off smaller ones. With time, the electrical circuits become "wiry" and excitable. Normally

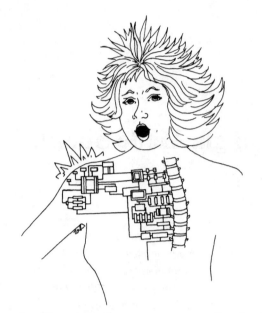

Fig. 2. *Cross-circuiting giving the wrong message after shoulder trauma.*

non-painful stimuli are regarded as painful ones. The "output" wires fail to alleviate discomfort. The circuits discharge signals that increase your perception of pain, not only in the region that was hurt but also in the area around it. As a result, the processes that regulate your body become confused and you start to develop all sorts of troublesome symptoms. You can't get a good night's sleep, your muscles go into spasm, and you become fatigued. This aggravates you further and creates a vicious cycle that makes the pain even worse. In a nutshell, this series of events is observed in fibromyalgia.

Let's explore how this happens and what can be done about it.

Part I

THE WHYS AND WHEREFORES OF FIBROMYALGIA

Is it nothing to you, all that pass by? Behold and see. Is there any pain like unto my pain, which is done unto me, wherewith the Lord has afflicted me in the day of his fierce anger? From above, he has sent fire into my bones.... and I am weary and faint all the day.

Jeremiah, in Lamentations 11:12–13

In this part the reader will discover how fibromyalgia evolved and was ultimately defined. Although descriptions of it date back to biblical times, the perception of fibromyalgia as a syndrome represents a convergence of two historical threads: those relating to ongoing musculoskeletal pain (joint and muscle aches) and those dealing with chronic fatigue and a sense of debility. Both official and practical definitions of fibromyalgia will be discussed, and we will consider the number of people who have the syndrome, as well as population groups that most frequently develop it.

1

How Our Understanding of Fibromyalgia Evolved

...and wearisome nights are appointed to me. When I lie down, I say, When shall I arise, and the night be gone? And I am full of tossings to and fro unto the dawning of the day...and the days of affliction have taken hold upon me. My bones are pierced in me in the night season; and my sinews take no rest.

Job 7:3–4 and 30:16–17.

There are times when rheumatologists have been accused of making up new syndromes. For example, in the last 40 years, our specialty has described new rheumatic entities including Lyme disease, the musculoskeletal manifestations of acquired immune deficiency syndrome (AIDS), eosinophilic-myalgia syndrome (from L-tryptophan contamination), and siliconosis (which, if it exists, results from silicone breast implants). Fibromyalgia is not in this group. Evidence for the syndrome can be found as far back in history as the book of Job, where he complained of "sinews (that) take no rest."

Concepts of what is now regarded as fibromyalgia date to the Babylonian epic of Gilgamesh, the Bible, and Shakespeare (*Therefore the moon, the governess of floods. Pale in her anger; washes the air. That rheumatic diseases do abound. A Midsummer Night's Dream, Act 2, Scene 34, I, 105*). The term "rheumatism" was first used by Guillaume de Baillou around 1592 and was included in a 1763 glossary of rheumatic diseases by FB de Sauvages de la Croix.

Fibromyalgia represents a convergence of concepts, as shown in Table 1.1. In other words, a similar clinical presentation ultimately evolved, and by the late 20th century it was apparent that these musculoskeletal manifestations of central pain or sensory augmentation represented a similar process.

EVOLUTION OF TRIGGER AND TENDER POINTS

The British physician RP Player first described what are now regarded as tender points in 1821 and were described in more detail by F Villeix in an 1841 treatise ("*points douloureaux*"). Additional insights derived in the 19th century include its predilection for females, the presence of nodules, associated muscular spasm,

Table 1.1. *Fibromyalgia: A Convergence of Concepts*

Trigger and tender points
Neurasthenia
Postinfectious fatigue syndromes
Chronic widespread pain in wartime
Myalgic encephalomyelitis
Myasthenic syndrome
Post-traumatic myofascial pain
"Continuous" trauma

pain and stiffness, and somatic complaints. Sir William R Gowers (1845–1915) coined the term "fibrositis" in a paper on lumbago (low back pain) in 1904. Sir Thomas Lewis and Jonas Kellgren mapped out tender and trigger points as well as referred pain patterns in the 1930s. Arthur Steindler demonstrated amelioration of local symptoms with procaine injections in 1937. Janet Travell (1901–1997) was the White House physician to John F Kennedy and Lyndon B Johnson. She elaborated upon these findings and is felt to be largely responsible for founding the discipline now known as physical medicine. In part because of a differing philosophy regarding the underlying pathophysiology, there has been a gradual divergence between what the terms tender point (an area of the body that displays increased tenderness upon palpation—the number of which is an (albeit poor) measure of an individual's overall pain sensitivity) and trigger point (a regional phenomenon accompanied by the presence of "taut bands" and referred pain) have come to mean.

NEURASTHENIA

The term "nervous exhaustion" or chronic fatigue was first studied by Austin Flint in the early 1800s and detailed by George Beard (1839–1883), who coined the term "neurasthenia" and Silas Weir Mitchell (1829–1914), who "packaged" the condition in the United States and treated it with a combination of Faradic currents and misogynistic approaches (e.g., removal of the clitoris, encouraging masturbation via horseback riding). Neurasthenia was the longest section in the 1899 edition of Sir William Osler's textbook of medicine. The term largely disappeared after World War I.

POST-INFECTIOUS FATIGUE SYNDROMES

The association between established infections and psychological or fatigue states was attributed to malaria or "wasting fevers" in the 1860s and typhoid fever by Osler among others. In the 1930s and 1940s, reports of post infectious fatigue syndromes were published relating to polio and brucellosis. In the 1970s, chronic fatigue was attributed to yeast and the Epstein-Barr virus, but rigorous study methods suggested that this either did not occur or was not limited to these microbes. Ultimately, terminology used by infectious disease and internal medicine specialists was refined by the Centers for Disease Control in their 1988 classification for defining cases of "chronic fatigue syndrome".

CHRONIC WIDESPREAD PAIN IN WARTIME

Complaints of chronic fatigue or musculoskeletal pain in wartime date back to the 1700s but were first documented by British pensioners after the Crimean War (1853–1856). "Effort syndrome" or "irritable heart" was noted by Jacob da Costa, a Union surgeon during the United States Civil War (1861–1865) where fatigue, difficulty sleeping, palpitations, digestive disturbances and headache required removal from the battlefield. Six hundred thousand cases of "da Costa's syndrome" were noted by the British military during the first World War (1914–1918). In 1942, 69% of all referrals to British military hospitals were for "fibrositis," which also included difficulty in carrying weaponry. Post-traumatic stress disorder (PTSD) was associated with musculoskeletal complaints by soldiers in the United States military during the Vietnam War (1961–1975) and Iraq conflicts (2003–2011). Post-war somatic syndromes are not confined to wars that are accompanied by intensely stressful events; in the first Gulf War there was very little PTSD but still a very high rate of post-deployment chronic widespread pain, fatigue, memory difficulties, etc.

MYALGIC ENCEPHALOMYELITIS

Also known as epidemic neuromyasthenia, the English terminology myalgic encephalomyelitis was applied to "outbreaks" of fibromyalgia after polio or other infectious epidemics between 1934 and 1987. Sometimes the onset of these events was associated with mass hysteria; chronicity of symptoms was a common feature.

MYASTHENIC SYNDROME

Before rheumatology was a recognized subspecialty and access to a rheumatology consultant was generally available, many individuals with fibromyalgia were diagnosed by neurologists between 1930 and 1965 as having "myasthenic syndrome," or myasthenic gravis-like symptoms with a negative Tensilon test. Interestingly, many of these patients were prescribed pyridostigmine with favorable responses, which led investigators at the University of Oregon to report that this agent had similar effects to growth hormone.

POST-TRAUMATIC MYOFASCIAL PAIN

In 1866, London surgeon John E Erichsen (1818–1896) described "Railway Spine" as a form of post-traumatic back pain that was more severe and of longer duration than expected from the attributable injury (Figure 1.1). A Los Angeles orthopedist, HD Crowe, described eight cases of post-automobile accident neck pain in 1928 and coined the term "whiplash." (Dr. Crowe went on to become a founding member of the Sierra Club). Widespread chronic musculoskeletal pain was reported in some of those cases. Legal considerations have made it difficult to separate science from fact in this area, but these patients have been shown to have widespread tenderness and hyperalgesia just as is seen in fibromyalgia.

"CONTINUOUS TRAUMA" AND FIBROMYALGIA

Myofascial pain among Welsh coal miners stemming from repeated heavy lifting was officially recognized by the British government as a compensable injury in

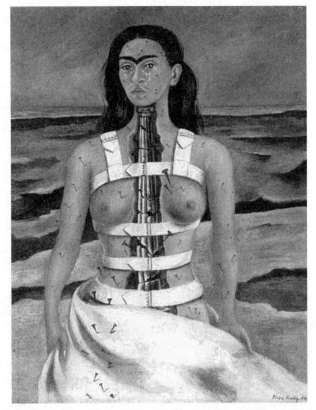

Fig. 1.1. *Reproduced from Arthritis Rheumatism 2000; 43: 708, with permission Frida Kahlo: The Broken Column (1916). Kahlo painted numerous self-portraits expressing the chronic pain she suffered subsequent to a bus accident. Reproduced with permission from Museo Delores Olmedo Patino, Mexico, City, Mexico.*

the 1920s as "Worker's Compensation" insurance plans were becoming wide-spread. This phenomenon was subject to considerable abuse as exemplified by the "epidemic" of "repetitive strain syndrome" among Australian workers in the 1980s that occurred and then largely disappeared when regulatory terminology was changed. Pre-employment psychological profiles and musculoskeletal complaints may play a role in predicting which employees with certain job descriptions will develop symptoms and seek compensation for their plight. The role of continuous trauma is nevertheless a real one and many of these individuals develop fibromyalgia.

SUMMING UP: THE CONVERGENCE OF CONCEPTS

Work in the 1970s by Hugh Smythe and colleagues at the University of Toronto connected the musculoskeletal complaints with poor sleep habits and tender points. Muhammad Yunus and colleagues at the University of Illinois in the 1980s renamed fibrositis as fibromyalgia and associated the above with somatic complaints and other functional syndromes. This led the American Medical Association to editorialize that fibromyalgia syndrome represented a distinct entity in 1987. An ad hoc committee of the American College of Rheumatology formulated and validated criteria for fibromyalgia syndrome in 1990, and the concept was endorsed by the Copenhagen declaration of the World Health Organization in 1992.

FOR FURTHER READING

Bennett RM, Fibromyalgia, *J American Medical Association* 1987; *257*: 2802–2803.

Smythe H, Fibrositis syndrome: a historical perspective. *J Rheumatology* 1989; *16*: (supp 19) 2–6.

Wallace DJ, Fibromyalgia: Unusual historical aspects and new pathogenetic insights, *Mt Sinai J Med.* 1984; *51*: 124–131.

Wallace DJ, The history of fibromyalgia. In: Wallace DJ and Clauw SJ, *eds. Fibromyalgia and Other Central Pain Syndromes.* Philadelphia, PA: Lippincott Williams & Wilkins; 2005; 1–8.

2

What Is Fibromyalgia?

A woman armed with sick headaches, nervousness, debility, presentiments, fears, horrors, and all sorts of imaginary and real diseases has an external armory of weapons of subjugation.

Harriet Beecher Stowe (1811–1896),
Pink and White Tyranny, 1871

When the Arthritis Foundation tried to categorize the 150 different forms of musculoskeletal conditions in 1963, it created a classification known as *soft tissue rheumatism*. Included in this listing are conditions in which joints are *not* involved. Soft tissue rheumatism encompasses the supporting structures of joints (e.g., ligaments, bursae, and tendons), muscles, and other soft tissues. Fibromyalgia is a form of soft tissue rheumatism. A combination of three terms—*fibro* (from the Latin *fibra,* or fibrous tissue), *myo-* (the Greek prefix *myos,* for muscles), and *algia* (from the Greek *algos,* which denotes pain)—fibromyalgia replaces earlier names for the syndrome that are still used by doctors and other health professionals such as *myofibrositis, myofascitis, muscular rheumatism, fibrositis,* and *generalized musculoligamentous strain*. Fibromyalgia is *not* a form of arthritis, since it is not associated with joint inflammation.

THE AMERICAN COLLEGE OF RHEUMATOLOGY (ACR) FIBROMYALGIA CRITERIA

In the late 1980s, a Multicenter Criteria Committee under the direction of Dr. Frederick Wolfe at the University of Kansas was formed to define fibromyalgia. In their study, 293 patients with presumed fibromyalgia were compared with 265 patients who had other rheumatic diseases in 16 centers throughout North America. The groups were evaluated for a variety of symptoms, signs, and laboratory abnormalities in an effort to ascertain which factors were the most *sensitive* and *specific* for defining the disorder. In other words, the investigators wanted to identify the most frequently found features of fibromyalgia (sensitivity) that could help doctors differentiate it from other disorders (specificity). The list in Table 2.1 (illustrated in Fig. 2.1) was 88.4% sensitive and 81.1% specific in identifying fibromyalgia patients. As a result, these criteria were endorsed in 1990 by the American College of Rheumatology (ACR), the association to which nearly all 5,000 rheumatologists in the United States and Canada belong.

Focusing on Table 2.1 and Figure 2.1, fibromyalgia essentially is:

1. Widespread pain of at least three months' duration (this rules out viruses or traumatic insults which resolve on their own).
2. Pain in all four quadrants of the body (picture cutting the body into quarters, as in a pie): right side, left side, above the waist, below the waist.
3. Pain occurring in at least 11 of 18 specified "tender" points (as shown in the figure) with at least one point in each quadrant.
4. Pain defined, in this context, as discomfort when eight pounds of pressure are applied to the tender point.

Tender points usually occur in a specific distribution. For instance, 8 of the 18 tender points are in the upper back and neck area, and only two are below the buttocks. The reader should be aware that tender points can occur almost anywhere in the body; the ACR criteria simply represent the most common 18 points. A consensus conference later agreed that the four factors listed above do not have to be present at the same time in order to meet the criteria. Therefore, a

Table 2.1. *The 1990 ACR Criteria for Fibromyalgia*

---

1. *History of widespread pain.*

Definition: Pain is considered widespread when all of the following are present: pain in the left side of the body, pain in the right side of the body, pain above the waist, and pain below the waist. In addition, axial skeletal pain (cervical spine or anterior chest or thoracic spine or low back) must be present. In this definition shoulder and buttock pain is considered as pain for each involved side. "Low back" pain is considered lower segment pain.

2. *Pain in 11 of 18 tender point sites on digital palpation.*

Definition: Pain, on digital palpation, must be present in at least 11 of the following 18 tender point sites:

Occiput: bilateral, at the suboccipital muscle insertions.

Low cervical: bilateral, at the anterior aspects of the inter-transverse spaces at C5–C7.

Trapezius: bilateral, at the midpoint of the upper border.

Supraspinatus: bilateral, at origins, above the scapula spine near the medial border.

2nd rib: bilateral, at the second costochondral junctions, just lateral to the junctions on upper surfaces.

Lateral epicondyle: bilateral, 2 cm distal to the epicondyles.

Gluteal: bilateral, in upper outer quadrants of buttocks in anterior fold of muscle.

Greater trochanter: bilateral, posterior to the trochanteric prominence.

Knees: bilateral, at the medial fat pad proximal to the joint line.

For a tender point to be considered "positive," the subject must state that the palpation was painful. "Tender" is not to be considered painful.

Note: For classification purposes patients will be said to have fibromyalgia if both criteria are satisfied.

Widespread pain must have been present for at least 3 months. The presence of a second clinical disorder does not exclude the diagnosis of fibromyalgia.

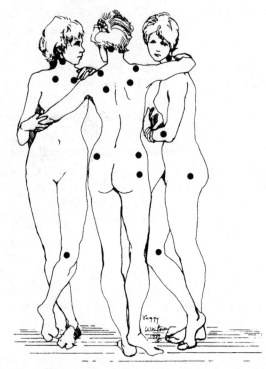

Fig. 2.1. *Fibromyalgia tender points. (Adapted from "The Three Graces," Louvre Museum, Paris. From D.J. Wallace, The Lupus Book. New York: Oxford University Press, 1995, p. 170; reprinted with permission from Dr. F. Wolfe.)*

patient may have only right buttock pain on one day and left upper back pain on another, or have different tender points on different days.

Once fibromyalgia was defined, it was possible to perform more reliable studies on this syndrome, since all researchers would be using the same definition. We could now explore how many people in the United States had fibromyalgia, determine what their primary complaints were, and identify groups of people on whom to test new treatments. Reporting a reproducible set of symptoms and signs has had additional fringe benefits: patients can be clearly educated on their condition; medical and other professional schools can teach students about fibromyalgia using a core terminology that has high sensitivity and specificity; and insurance companies now recognize fibromyalgia as a distinct syndrome.

OTHER FEATURES OF FIBROMYALGIA

In the previous chapter, we mentioned that fibromyalgia is associated with fatigue, sleep disturbances, and bowel complaints, among other symptoms and signs. How do these symptoms fit into the definition of fibromyalgia? The criteria committee considered these findings and correlated them statistically with the syndrome, but the symptoms did not have a high enough score in enough patients to be part of the definition. For example, Dr. Wolfe, in another article in 1990, stated that sleep disturbance, fatigue, numbness or tingling, and anxiety had more than a 60% occurrence in defining fibromyalgia, and headache or irritable bowel had more than a 50% occurrence. In fact, he observed that the presence of seven of 18 tender points with four of the six features listed above was "highly suspicious" for the diagnosis.

In response to this, a group of international fibromyalgia experts issued what was termed the Copenhagen Declaration in 1992, which was adopted by the World Health Organization in 1993. They recognized the use of the ACR criteria for research purposes but defined fibromyalgia as being part of a wider spectrum encompassing headache, irritable bladder, spastic colitis, painful menstrual periods, temperature sensitivity, atypical patterns of numbness and tingling, exercise intolerance, and complaints of weakness in addition to persistent fatigue, stiffness, and nonrestoring sleep.

FIBROMYALGIA TERMINOLOGY: CLASSIFICATION AND REGIONAL FORMS

Many rheumatologists recognize two types of fibromyalgia: primary and secondary. The cause of *primary fibromyalgia syndrome* is unknown, but it can be induced by trauma, infection, stress, inflammation, or other factors. *Secondary fibromyalgia* occurs when a primary condition, such as hypothyroidism or lupus, creates a concomitant fibromyalgia, the treatment of which may make the syndrome disappear. The next chapter will review this topic in more detail.

Sometimes, pain identical to that associated with fibromyalgia is located in specific areas or regions or in one quadrant of the body. For example, patients may have jaw and neck pain on one side and no discomfort anywhere else. Regional forms of fibromyalgia are called *regional myofascial syndrome* or *myofascial pain syndrome*. This entity is reviewed in detail in chapter 12.

Finally, patients may hear a lot about trigger points or tender points. Many doctors consider them to be the same thing. However, for research purposes, there are subtle differences. A *tender point* is an area of tenderness in the muscles, tendons, bony prominences, or fat pads, whereas a *trigger point* shoots down to another area. For instance, when a trigger point is touched, it shoots pain to other muscles. Like pulling a trigger in a gun, it sends out a bullet that travels, and pain can be felt in areas away from the trigger.

HOW TO RESPOND TO PEOPLE WHO DO NOT BELIEVE FIBROMYALGIA EXISTS

Since fibromyalgia is a relatively new entity, some physicians who may have had the topic barely covered in medical school tend to downplay its importance; they may say "its all psychiatric," or deny its existence. Many training programs are almost entirely hospital-based and few patients with fibromyalgia are ever hospitalized for it. Most importantly, fibromyalgia is not a *disease*; it is a *syndrome* or a *construct*. Simply stated, fibromyalgia is a form of *chronic widespread pain* that meets statistically validated criteria. Some doctors don't like the name "fibromyalgia" because it could stigmatize patients. Since the syndrome encompasses individuals with lupus, scoliosis, and hypothyroidism, fibromyalgia's boundaries tend to defy the occasional patient's desire to blame the syndrome as the reason why they cannot work, function in society, or be happy. The authors have heard fibromyalgia being called *the Emperor's new clothes syndrome, generalized rheumatism,* or *feeling out of sorts.* Nevertheless, every recognized medical organization from the American College of Rheumatology, the American Medical Association, the World Health Organization, and the American College of Physicians to medical insurers have endorsed its existence. There has never been a published peer-review study or report from a medical society challenging the validity of fibromyalgia as a syndrome or construct. Finally, some critics refuse to recognize fibromyalgia as an entity because it lacks firm physical signs. Not only is this not the case, but the same analogy applies to migraine headaches. Nobody disputes the existence of migraines, and Americans spend $20 billion a year on their treatment.

Failings and Misuse of the 1990 Criteria Led to a Modified Revision

There were many problems with the ACR criteria, especially when they are misused and applied to individual patients in clinical practice. These include:

- They assume that the pain threshold for women and men are similar, and thus use the same threshold of 11 tender points as being indicative of fibromyalgia in both women and men. In fact, women are much more sensitive to pain, using any type of experimental pain testing, than men. Thus we should either apply greater pressure or accept lower numbers of tender points to consider a male tender, and this would lead to more males being appropriately diagnosed with fibromyalgia.
- We now know that fibromyalgia patients are more tender throughout the entire body, not just in these 18 locations. In fact, we now know that tender points are merely areas of the body where anyone is more tender. The difference between the pain threshold of a fibromyalgia patient and a control is just as great in areas such as the thumbnail and forehead as in regions considered to be tender points, so one can push anywhere in the body to assess pain threshold.
- Tender points are not a good measure of pressure pain threshold, since the number of tender points an individual displays is in part related to their pain threshold, and in part related to distress levels. More sophisticated measures of experimental pain or sensory testing are far superior to counting tender points in assessing an individual's overall pain or sensory threshold.

Also, although the criteria have been validated by other surveys, the ACR classification focused only upon pain. It ignores important FM symptoms such as fatigue, cognitive disturbance, alterations in sleep architecture and psychological distress as well as commonly associated syndromes such as irritable bowel syndrome. Further, the legal community has taken a narrow view of the criteria in applying it to litigation which ignores considerations enumerated in the beginning of this paragraph. As a result, Dr. Wolfe and his colleagues undertook to improve upon the 1990 effort.

THE 2010 AMERICAN COLLEGE OF RHEUMATOLOGY CRITERIA REVISION

This multicenter center study of 829 previously diagnosed FM patients took into account the above criticisms and expanded the diagnostic variables to include a widespread pain index (WPI) and categorical scales for cognitive symptoms, unrefreshed sleep, fatigue, and a number of body symptoms. A severity index was proposed which allows for longitudinal evaluation of patients. It is demonstrated in Table 2.2. This new metric can be used along with or instead of the 1990 criteria and is over 90% sensitive and specific.

OTHER FIBROMYALGIA RELATED CONSTRUCTS:

Chronic Widespread Pain

A highly respected epidemiologic unit in Manchester, United Kingdom addressed some of the failings of the ACR criteria and was concerned that cases of clinically meaningful widespread pain could be excluded. Their definition of "chronic widespread pain" differs from the ACR "four quadrant" one in that it requires more diffuse limb pain, present in two or more sections of contralateral limbs, and axial pain present for three months. These individuals have more severe disability and higher levels of associated symptoms. Chronic widespread pain can also often be present without tender points.

Table 2.2. *2010 Preliminary ACR Diagnostic Criteria for Fibromyalgia (FM)*

FM can be diagnosed based on a questionnaire administered by a health care professional if all three conditions are met:
1. Widespread pain index (WPI): The number of painful body regions (Scored 0–19 where the patient has had pain over the previous week with a score of at least 5)
2. Symptom severity scale that assesses fatigue, waking unrefreshed, cognitive symptoms, and quantifies the occurrence of other somatic symptoms. Each category is rated on a 0–3 scale with a final score of 0–12. The somatic symptom category includes over 20 complaints including muscle pain, numbness, tingling, depression, dry mouth, bladder spasm, etc.
3. Pain and symptoms present for 3 months or longer with no other disorder to explain it.

F Wolfe et al, Arthritis Care Res 2010; 62: 600–610

Regional Myofascial Pain (Myofascial Pain Syndrome)

There is considerable controversy regarding the existence of myofascial pain as a discrete entity. On one end of the continuum are many who feel that myofascial pain may be a pathophysiology distinct from fibromyalgia, and represent a local muscle process. At the other end of the continuum are others (including the authors) who feel that in many or even most cases, myofascial pain is merely a regional form of fibromyalgia. Regional myofascial pain patients tend to include more males and be more work or repetitive task related.

We will not try to resolve this controversy, but would suggest that patients with myofascial pain may respond well to the therapies suggested for fibromyalgia, and conversely, if a patient has primarily regional pain and does not display more "systemic" features such as diffuse tenderness, fatigue, memory problems, pain elsewhere in the body, that these individuals may benefit from local therapies that have been shown to be of value in myofascial pain. Also, since we know that a significant minority of patients with regional pain can develop widespread pain (likely via processes such as central sensitization) it is important to treat regional pain aggressively to attempt to prevent this from occurring.

Central Sensitivity Syndromes

Central sensitivity syndromes (CSS) is a term coined by Yunus that includes all syndromes characterized by failure to adequately dampen sensory afferent signals with a resultant amplification of pain. Although this term has not gained wide acceptance, the underlying construct is the same as that proposed by advocates of terms such as "functional somatic syndromes," somatization, chronic multisymptom illnesses, medically unexplained syndromes, etc.

The reason we prefer to use the term CSS in this book is that at present this term seems to give the most accurate information regarding the underlying pathophysiology of these illnesses. Nearly all of the conditions within this spectrum have been characterized by hypersensitivity to pain, e.g., performing experimental pain testing and identifying widespread hyperalgesia (increased pain to normally non-painful stimuli) and allodynia (pain in response to normally non-painful stimuli). In most of these conditions there are also data suggesting a more global problem with hypersensitivity to any type of sensory stimuli, and we are beginning to understand the neurobiology of this phenomenon (and the neurobiology is independent of psychological factors). Most patients with FM have a personal history of at least one and usually more of these associated syndromes, and these conditions are very familial and genetic, so it is common to see individuals whose family members have a history of regional and widespread pain (see Chapter 4 for pathogenesis). These entities can be regional or systemic and are listed in Table 2.3.

Table 2.3. *Examples of Some Central Sensitization Syndromes*

Fibromyalgia
Myofascial pain syndrome
Temporomandibular disorder
Whiplash
Repetitive strain disorder
Chronic idiopathic low back pain
Chronic fatigue syndrome; postinfectious fatigue syndromes
Gastrointestinal syndromes
Non-ulcer dyspepsia
Esophageal dysmotility
Irritable bowel syndrome
Biliary dyskinesia; post cholecystectomy syndrome
Cardiac region syndromes
Syndrome X
Non-cardiac chest pain
Costochrondritis
Mitral valve prolapse
Headache: tension-type, migraine
Gynecologic syndromes
Primary dysmenorrhea
Chronic pelvic pain
Dyspareunia, vulvodynia, vulvar vestibulitis
Endometriosis
Urologic syndromes
Irritable bladder/painful bladder
Interstitial cystitis
Chronic prostatitis
Psychiatric conditions
Depression/anxiety
Post-traumatic stress disorder
Bipolar illness
Obsessive compulsive disorder
Multiple chemical sensitivities (a form of anxiety)
Periodic limb movement disorder
Dysautonomias

OUTDATED TERMINOLOGY

The following terms have been used historically to describe some of the above conditions but no longer have any meaningful validity: myofasciitis, fibrositis, neurasthenia, myalgic encephalomyelitis, and myositis with normal muscle enzyme levels.

SUMMING UP

The term *fibromyalgia* refers to a complex syndrome characterized by pain amplification, musculoskeletal discomfort, and systemic symptoms. Although its existence was questioned in the past, nearly all rheumatologists, medical societies, and the overwhelming majority of physicians now accept fibromyalgia as a distinct diagnostic entity. Individuals who eventually develop fibromyalgia often have a history of other regional syndromes that fall under the umbrella of "central sensitivity syndromes." Recent evidence suggests that there is neurobiological evidence of pain and sensory amplification in these disorders. In addition, prominent psychological, social, and cognitive factors play a role in symptom expression in these illnesses. An understanding of the confluence of factors that can lead to symptom expression gives the underpinning for an effective management strategy for these patients.

FOR FURTHER READING

Csillag C. Fibromyalgia: the Copenhagen Declaration. *Lancet 340*, 1992: 663–664.

MacFarlane GJ, Croft PR, Schollum J, *et al.* Widespread pain: Is an improved classification possible? *J Rheumatol* 1996; *23*: 1628–1632.

Yunus MB, Central sensitivity syndromes: A new paradigm and group nosology for fibromyalgia and overlapping conditions, and the related issue of disease versus illness. *Seminars Arthritis Rheumatism* 2008; *37*: 339–352.

Yunus M, Masi AT, Calabro JJ, *et al.* Primary fibromyalgia (fibrositis): Clinical study of 50 patients with matched normal controls. *Seminars Arthritis Rheum 11*, 1981: 151–171.

Wolfe F, Smythe HA, Yunus MB, Bennett RM, *et al.* The American College of Rheumatology criteria for the classification of fibromyalgia. *Report of the multicenter criteria committee, Arthritis Rheum* 1990; *33*: 160–172.

Wolfe F, Clauw DJ, Fitzcharles M-A, The American College of Rheumatology Preliminary Diagnostic Criteria for Fibromyalgia and Measurement of Symptom Severity. *Arthritis Care & Research* 2010; *62*: 600–610.

3

Who Gets Fibromyalgia and Why?

I am glad my case is not serious but these nervous troubles are dreadfully depressing.

Charlotte Perkins Gilman (1860–1935),
The Yellow Wallpaper, 1913

When fibromyalgia is first diagnosed, patients often have two reactions. The first reaction is relief. They have a legitimate diagnosis and are not crazy. Then a feeling of loneliness and a hint of fear can be detected, since many patients have never heard of the fibromyalgia syndrome and do not know what to do. It is worth repeating that the intent of this book is to promote a better understanding of fibromyalgia, as well as to provide patients, allied health professionals, and physicians with ways to work together. But first, this chapter will discuss how many people have fibromyalgia and how it might have been acquired.

HOW PREVALENT IS FIBROMYALGIA?

Until recently, nobody knew how many people had fibromyalgia. Dr. Frederick Wolfe, the same physician who chaired the ACR Criteria Committee, received funding to undertake an epidemiologic survey of the syndrome. Using computerized applications of field methodologies to estimate the prevalence of fibromyalgia (the number of cases per 100,000 individuals), his team estimated that six million people in the United States fulfill the ACR criteria for fibromyalgia. This and other surveys suggest that while 2% of the adult U.S. population have full-blown fibromyalgia (3.5% of adult women and 0.5% of adult men), 11% have chronic widespread pain and 20% have chronic regional pain. Dr. Larry Bradley at the University of Alabama has found that for every diagnosed fibromyalgia patient in the United States, there is an undiagnosed individual who has the requisite tender points, but never seeks medical attention for this. This has been termed *community fibromyalgia.* A survey in Great Britain found that 13% of the population had chronic widespread pain, 72% of whom sought medical attention for it. Of those, 21% fulfilled the ACR criteria for fibromyalgia. In other words, of individuals with chronic neuromuscular pain, less than half have diagnosed fibromyalgia or community fibromyalgia. A 2012 survey by the Mayo Clinic demonstrated that in Olmstead County, Minnesota, among those diagnosed by a health care provider and mail survey the prevalence was 1.1% and 6.4% respectively. Figure 3.1 summarizes where fibromyalgia comes from.

Fibromyalgia is the third or fourth most common reason for consulting a rheumatologist. Approximately 15 to 20% of all patients seeking rheumatology referrals have fibromyalgia. Prevalence estimates vary widely depending of methods of ascertainment. This could be a postal survey, health plan coding inventory, and hospital discharge diagnosis or clinic population. For example, one epidemiologic survey concluded that 10% of Norwegians have FM, while another in neighboring Denmark found a prevalence figure of 0.66%. The 5,000 rheumatologists in the United States who are trained in internal medicine and subspecialize in managing more than 150 musculoskeletal and immune system disorders are very familiar with the diagnosis and treatment of fibromyalgia.

WHO DEVELOPS FIBROMYALGIA?

Even though one American in 50 has fibromyalgia, the syndrome is distributed unevenly across the population. Eighty to ninety percent of patients with the condition are women. (One theory contends that women have a lower pain threshold than men, which is hormonally related.) Fibromyalgia is extremely uncommon in children and rarely appears for the first time in older persons. Within these groups, complaints and clinical features are atypical (see Chapter 16). In the United States, fibromyalgia is more common among Caucasians than among other racial groups. Using the ACR criteria or other earlier suggested criteria, the prevalence of fibromyalgia in other countries or regions (mostly in Europe, Canada, and Australia) has ranged from 0.5% to 12%. Hence, there are probably at a minimum 5 million, and up to 15 million Americans with FM. Some researchers have observed an increased prevalence among first-generation immigrant families in the United States. For instance, our research group has been struck by the relatively high prevalence of fibromyalgia among recently arrived Iranians and Russians. In one survey, the prevalence of FM in professional workers was almost zero, 0.5% of those employed in industry, 0.8% of service workers, 1.5% in agriculture, and 1.9% of those never employed. Risk factors for developing FM include poor sleep, psychological distress, smoking, fatigue, anxiety, a family history of FM, and presence of any of the somatic associated symptoms.

Are humans the only species to develop fibromyalgia? Probably not. Lameness has been observed in dogs for some time, and articles in the veterinary literature convincingly show that they can also have tender points.

HOW OLD DO YOU HAVE TO BE TO GET FIBROMYALGIA?

Most of our fibromyalgia patients are in their prime of life and at the peak of their careers. Surveys have shown that most patients develop the syndrome in their 30s and 40s. Fibromyalgia infrequently evolves during adolescence. Whereas 60% of cases are diagnosed in people between the ages of 30 and 49, another 35% of patients are diagnosed in their 20s or between the age of 50 and 65. The reasons for this distribution are not clear, but the decline in onset after the age of 50 may have something to do with menopause in women, which may alleviate (but occasionally aggravate) certain fibromyalgia symptoms.

IS FIBROMYALGIA GENETIC?

In the mid-1980s, one research study suggested that fibromyalgia patients had an increased prevalence of a specific gene. These results, however, were shown to be inaccurate when confirmatory studies were performed on a larger scale. Even though no fibromyalgia genetic markers have been found, we are aware of studies documenting a high prevalence of the syndrome among certain families and evidence that a portion of pain perception is genetically mediated. Certain pain amplification genes may play a role as well (Chapter 4). For example, in one well-documented study, 28% of the children of fibromyalgia patients ultimately developed the syndrome. Whether this is due to a yet-undiscovered genetic marker or markers, or from environmental or psychological factors is still unclear.

WHAT ARE SOME OF THE CAUSES OF FIBROMYALGIA?

What turns on the fibromyalgia syndrome? The biology, chemistry, hormonal factors, and immune factors involved are detailed in Part II of this book. However, when we ask patients what they feel caused their fibromyalgia, trauma, infections, and stress are the three most common responses.

Fibromyalgia Resulting from a Single-Event Trauma

Becky was enjoying the feel of her brand-new roadster when somebody who wasn't paying attention rear-ended her at 10 miles per hour while she was stopped at a red light. The bumper was dented, and so was Becky's future. A day later, she began to complain of stiffness . aching in her upper back and neck, along with headaches. She was initially diagnosed on the basis of a stiff neck as having a whiplash injury. Dr. Allen treated her with ibuprofen, a soft neck collar, and a mild muscle relaxant. When she failed to improve, physical therapy was prescribed a week later. Over the next three months, Becky's pain spread to her lower back, legs, and elbows.

She could no longer sleep through the night. The pain worsened as the day progressed or if the weather changed. Her skin became sensitive to the touch, particularly if the physical therapist worked her too hard. Dr. Allen diagnosed her as having post-traumatic fibromyalgia and initiated a specific treatment program.

When we last counted, there were 47 different reported secondary causes of fibromyalgia. *According to patients,* the most common cause of secondary fibromyalgia is trauma. There are two types of trauma: injury resulting from a single event or continuous trauma with resulting repetitive injury.

First, let's discuss a single-event injury. Suppose that in your community 100 people sustain a whiplash injury from a 10-mile-per-hour rear-ender automobile accident on a given day. "Whiplash," a term coined by H. D. Crowe in 1928, is the only diagnosis relating to causation rather than the tissue involved. A whiplash injury occurs when a car driver or passenger is rear-ended. The head and neck stay still at first, while the body jerks forward. As the body returns back, the neck hyperextends backward. What happens to people after a whiplash injury? Many will go to their doctor within days and report pain in their upper back and neck areas. Their doctor will prescribe ibuprofen or naproxen-like anti-inflammatory agents, a muscle relaxant, and perhaps even a small prescription for a strong painkiller. A minority may be given a neck collar or physical or chiropractic therapy. After two-three months, all but two to five percent (up to 21% in some studies) of the patients will get better and gradually discontinue all therapy. But what about the remaining people? Strange things start to happen. For completely unclear reasons, these two to five percent begin to hurt more and their pain becomes widespread. They complain of lower back and leg pain (areas that were not injured), begin noticing difficulty sleeping, and become fatigued. Ultimately, they are diagnosed as having fibromyalgia. Many doctors don't understand this; they suffered the same trivial injury with the same impact from which other patients fully recover! We have seen this with slip-and-fall injuries and other forms of minor trauma. This phenomenon is poorly documented in the medical literature, and since litigation frequently is involved, many doctors feel it is overdiagnosed.

Physical trauma is undisputedly associated with post-event localized pain. In some individuals, this regional pain fails to resolve and in fact becomes more widespread and chronic. The rate at which regional pain syndromes such as whiplash convert to chronic widespread pain differs markedly from country to country. Although it would be appealing to assume that these differences are due to differences in disability and litigation systems within different countries, this does not seem to be the case, as this occurs commonly in countries with "no fault" and/or national health insurance. Unfortunately, controversy regarding these social and political issues regarding litigation and compensation often distract clinicians, and they "throw out the baby with the bathwater," ignoring the overwhelming data that "FM is real" because they do not feel patients are "worthy" of being eligible for these processes.

The authors wish to emphasize a few points:

a. 90% of post-traumatic myofascial pain resolves within three months if there is no serious injury (e.g., fracture, shock).
b. A review of a patient's prior medical record or history in those who claim new onset of myofascial pain or FM often reveals evidence of a central sensitization syndrome in the overwhelming majority, although it may not have been labeled as such. The court system can decide whether this is still a compensable injury in this setting.
c. True post-traumatic FM should only be considered when there is a close temporal relationship between regional pain that is due to trauma, and the subsequent development of more widespread pain.
d. Long-standing, chronic widespread pain with tender points (FM) after a trivial injury may occur but is extremely rare.
e. A pre-existing fibromyalgia or myofascial pain syndrome can be aggravated by trauma and many other types of stress.

Fibromyalgia from Continuous Trauma

Although Jared was found to have scoliosis as a child, it did not interfere with his activities or lifestyle. After graduating from junior college, he took a job as a shipping clerk. His responsibilities included preparing packages for delivery that weighed up to 50 pounds and carrying them to the loading dock. Jared also had to log the shipment's specifications onto the company's computer and track when they were sent and received. After six weeks on the job, Jared started to notice discomfort in his upper and lower back and experienced occasional numbness in his left hand. At first, naproxen (Aleve) relieved the symptoms, and he noted that the pain diminished on weekends. After three months on the job, Jared was barely able to make it to work. A family physician gave him a muscle relaxant and a few hydrocodone bitartrate/acetaminophen (Vicodin) to take for severe pain and prescribed physical therapy. He felt better after the therapy sessions, but relief did not last. His family physician referred Jared to an orthopedist, who requested an occupational therapy evaluation. Ginger, the therapist, closely scrutinized how Jared lifted boxes and supported his weight in relation to his scoliosis and the company's holding tables. She also watched how Jared sat and functioned when he worked at the computer. Ginger recommended that he wear a lumbar band at work, taught him how to straddle his weight, and adjusted the height and back of the computer chair. Jared was instructed in strengthening exercises, and the computer monitor's angle was altered. Jared now takes only Aleve occasionally and is largely pain free.

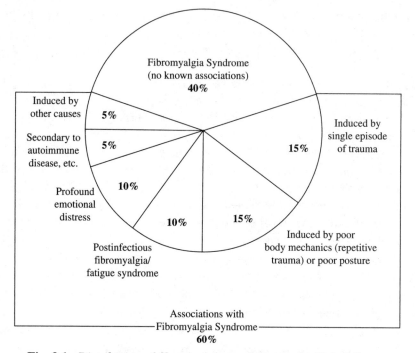

Fig. 3.1. *Distribution of fibromyalgia syndrome in the United States.*

Jared's complaints are extremely common. Repetitive trauma from poor work-station body mechanics (usually associated with regional myofascial syndrome) is especially common among workers who do heavy lifting. The legal term "continuous trauma" opens up another can of worms because it also involves litigation, particularly worker's compensation. Chapters 12 and 24 discuss repetitive strain syndrome and disability issues in more detail. Repetitive heavy lifting, pulling, bending, stooping, squatting, or strains (e.g., brought on by excessive keyboarding hand use) among other activities can lead to regional myofascial pain. If not adequately addressed, a small percentage of these individuals may evolve into FM. Unfortunately, these complaints are confounded when made part of a Worker's Compensation complaint by a variety of factors which are reviewed in Chapter 23.

What about Infections?

One of the most common self-reported causes of fibromyalgia is an infectious process, possibly a viral (e.g., an Epstein-Barr-like) illness characterized by fever, swollen glands, sore throat, and cough. When these conditions disappear, the patient develops profound aching and fatigue. Over 40 microbes have been associated with postinfectious fatigue syndromes and are reviewed in

Chapter 13. The inciting organisms are quite diverse and include parvovirus, the herpes virus causing mononucleosis and Epstein-Barr, mycoplasma, *Toxoplasma gondii,* hepatitis A virus, cytomegalovirus, *Brucella,* poliovirus, parvovirus, the virus causing AIDS, and the bacterium causing Lyme disease.

Inflammation or Medication-related FM

A relatively high percentage (e.g., up to 20%) of patients with inflammatory conditions such as rheumatoid arthritis or systemic lupus erythematosus develop FM. When this occurs patients need to be treated for both the inflammatory disease and the FM. Also, some anti-inflammatory regimens (e.g., corticosteroids, alpha-interferon) can produce hyperesthesia, aching, or cognitive changes associated with FM.

Psychological Stress and Distress

Although there is no question that psychological stress may sometimes trigger or exacerbate FM, not all "stress" seems to be equally capable of doing this, and not all people with "stress" develop chronic widespread pain (CWP) or FM. For example, population-based studies show that individuals with high levels of distress (but no pain) in the population are about twice as likely to develop CWP as those without distress. However, even though there is a higher relative risk, the overwhelming majority of new cases of CWP in the community *did not* have high levels of distress at baseline.

With respect to the type of stress that can best trigger or exacerbate these illnesses, it seems as though interpersonal stressors are the most likely. On the other hand, community stressors, such as the terrorists attacks of September 11, 2001, did not seem to lead to a higher rate of FM in the population of New York City, or worsen pre-existing FM in patients in Washington D.C.

Finally, patients with a history of nearly any type of psychiatric disorder have an increased likelihood of developing FM, and individuals with FM are also more likely to develop many types of psychiatric disorders. This is consistent with data showing a weak shared familial predisposition for psychiatric disorders and FM and related syndromes. This likely occurs because genetic abnormalities involving the breakdown or activity of neurotransmitters that are involved in both psychiatric disorders and pain (e.g., serotonin, norepinephrine, Substance P) lead to a higher rate of both types of disorders, and because stress can trigger both types of disorders.

This theoretical link between stress, changes in stress axis activity, and subsequent susceptibility to develop somatic symptoms or syndromes is also supported by studies showing that patients with fibromyalgia and related conditions may be more likely than non-affected individuals to have experienced physical or sexual abuse in childhood. Twin studies have recently supported a link between post-traumatic stress disorder (PTSD) and trauma, and CWP. A study of Israeli war veterans with PTSD showed that those who exercised regularly were much less likely to develop CWP or fibromyalgia.

SUMMING UP

At least 2% of the population of nearly any country or culture have FM. Most individuals presently diagnosed are women who were diagnosed in their 30s or 40s, but more males and younger individuals will be diagnosed as clinicians become more comfortable with making this diagnosis. While the inciting factor that brought on FM is often not known, stressors such as trauma, psychological distress, infections, inflammation, or medication can antedate many cases.

FOR FURTHER READING

Jones GT, Nicholl BJ, Mc Beth J, *et al.* Role of road traffic accidents and other traumatic events in the onset of chronic widespread pain: Results from a population-based prospective study, *Arthritis Care Res* 2011: *63*: 696–701.

Mc Lean S, Clauw DJ, Williams DA. The role of trauma in chronic neuromuscular pain, In Wallace DJ and Clauw DJ, *eds. Fibromyalgia and Other Central Pain Syndromes.* Philadelphia, PA: Lippincott Williams & Wilkins 2007; 267–279.

Vincent A, Lahr BD, Wolfe F, *et al.* Prevalence of fibromyalgia: A population-based study in Olmsted County, Minnesota, utilizing the Rochester Epidemiology project, *Arthritis Care Res* 2012; E pub Nov 30.

White KP, Speechley M, Harth M, *et al.* The London fibromyalgia epidemiology study: Comparing the demographic and clinical characteristics in 100 random community cases of fibromyalgia versus controls, *J Rheumatology* 1999; *26*: 885–889.

Wolfe F, Ross K, Anderson J, *et al.* The prevalence and characteristics of fibromyalgia in the general population, *Arthritis Rheum* 1995; *38*: 19–28.

Part II
BASIC SCIENCE AND FIBROMYALGIA

Pain is perfect misery, the worst of evils and excessive, overturns all patience.

John Milton (1608–1674),
Paradise Lost, 1667

The next four chapters discuss what makes fibromyalgia a *pain amplification syndrome.* We will first review the path normal pain takes and then relate why things might go awry in fibromyalgia. There are many candidates whose potential deviations will be evaluated. Abnormal connections between hormones, the immune system, sleep physiology, muscle pathology, and abnormalities of the nervous system are described. Unlike the rest of the book, this part uses a lot of technical language. Table 2 and the Glossary will help the reader navigate Part II successfully. You may wish to skip this part at this time and return to it later.

4

Why and How Do We Hurt?

When pain is unbearable it destroys us; when it does not it is bearable.
Marcus Aurelius (121–180),
Meditations vi, ca. 170 C.E.

A fibromyalgia patient frequently complains of pain. The pain of fibromyalgia is different from that of a headache, stomach cramp, toothache, or swollen joint. It has been described as a type of stiffness or aching, often associated with spasm. Unlike the other pains mentioned above, fibromyalgia pain responds poorly to aspirin, acetaminophen (Tylenol), or ibuprofen (Advil, Motrin). In fact, studies have suggested that even narcotics such as morphine are minimally beneficial if at all in ameliorating fibromyalgia pain. Why is it that fibromyalgia patients can take codeine, Vicodin, or even Dilaudid for musculoskeletal aches and have only a slight response? What produces "pain without purpose"?

In this chapter, we'll explore what makes fibromyalgia a pain amplification syndrome. Why does the patient hurt in places where there was often no injury and all laboratory tests are normal? What creates what doctors call *allodynia,* or a clinical situation that results in pain from a stimulus (such as light touch) that normally should *not* be painful? Fibromyalgia is a form of chronic, widespread allodynia, as well as sustained *hyperalgesia,* or greater sensitivity than would be expected to an adverse stimulus.

NORMAL PAIN PATHWAYS

The nervous system consists of several components. The brain and spinal cord comprise the *central nervous system.* Nerves leaving the spinal cord that tell us to move our arms or legs are part of the motor aspects of the *peripheral nervous system.* Additionally, all sorts of information about touch, taste, chemicals, and pressure are relayed through sensory pathways back to the spinal cord, where they are processed and sent up to the brain for a response. The *autonomic nervous system* consists of specialized peripheral nerves.

ACUTE VERSUS CHRONIC PAIN

Fibromyalgia is a disorder characterized by an inappropriate neuromuscular reaction that leads to chronic pain. Patients with fibromyalgia usually react normally to acute pain. Our current concepts of the way the body responds to chronic painful stimuli stem from the *gate theory,* first proposed by Ronald Melzack and Patrick Wall in 1965. Nerve "wires" go from the periphery to the dorsal horn of the spinal cord. These wires are modulated by feedback loops within the nervous system. Each wire ending, or "gate," may open or close in response to pain impulses. When large and small fibers carrying sensory signals arrive at the spinal cord at the same time, a "gate" opens. Structures in the lower part of the brain known as the *brain stem* receive notice of this input at the spinal cord level and signal it how to respond, and usually let the large fiber's package in first.

To elaborate upon this, nerve wires from the skin, muscles, or joints send sensory signals (e.g., touch, pressure) to the spinal cord. Several separate sensory pathways have been described. The particular sensory trail important in fibromyalgia is one termed *nociception.* A *nociceptor* is a receptor that is sensitive to a noxious stimulus. Nociceptors are present in blood vessel walls, muscle, fascia, tendons, joint capsules, fat pads, and on body surfaces. A noxious stimulus can be thermal (heat, cold), mechanical (touch, pressure), or chemical. Normally, the body transmits these nociceptive impulses neurochemically from the periphery to the central nervous system. *One factor that distinguishes acute from chronic pain is that the perception of chronic pain is significantly influenced by the interaction of physiologic, psychological, and social processes.* Unlike patients with acute pain, those with chronic pain often don't appear to be in pain. See Table 4.1.

Types of Wiring and Insulation: The Ascending Tract

All sorts of fibers make up the wires that connect the periphery to the spinal cord. Of the 3,000 nerve fibers in the ascending tract, some of the wires are quite heavy and insulated, while others are thin and unprotected. The nociceptive pathway is transmitted to the spinal cord by *unmyelinated* (uninsulated) *C fibers* and *myelinated* (insulated) *A-delta (Group 3)* fibers (Fig. 4.1). For example, unmyelinated C fibers carry diffuse, burning pain sensations, while myelinated A-delta fibers transmit signals from strong, noxious stimuli potentially damaging to tissues. Both also carry proprioceptive signals (balance, touch, and pressure). *B fibers* are myelinated nerves that are part of the autonomic nervous system. In a part of the spinal cord known as the *dorsal root ganglion,* a group of chemicals known as *neuropeptides* are released and travel up to the brain. Neuropeptides transmit nociceptive signals to spinal cord nerve cells and modulate (amplify or downgrade) the body's pain response. They

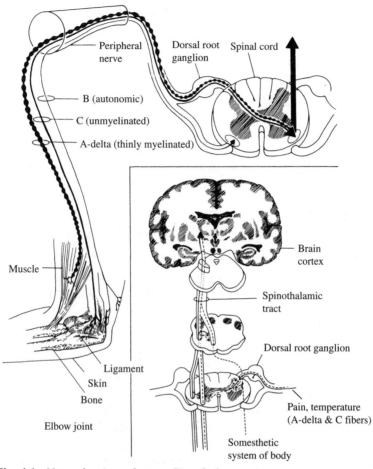

Fig. 4.1. *Normal pain pathways. Signals from pain receptors in muscles, joints, skin, ligaments, and bone are transmitted by A-delta and C fibers to the spinal cord. A-delta and C signals are sent to the thalamus of the brain via the spinothalamic tract after exiting the dorsal root ganglion, where neurotransmitters are released.*

have exotic names that only a neurophysiologist could be proud of, including, among others, *substance P, calcitonin-related gene peptide, nerve growth factor, norepinephrine, enkephalin-containing interneurons,* and *neurokinin A.* From the dorsal horn of the spinal cord, neuropeptides transmit information about the intensity and quality of the signal from the spine up to the thalamus of the brain via the *spinothalamic tract.* The thalamus interprets sensory and discriminative aspects of pain and sends messages further up the brain, which processes these signals and secretes a chemical known as an *endorphin,* which can mute or eliminate pain.

Table 4.1. *Pain Classifications Relevant to Fibromyalgia*

I. Acute pain—usually reacts normally in fibromyalgia
II.Chronic pain
  A.Psychogenic pain—not part of fibromyalgia
  B.Organic pain
    1. Location
      a. Localized—observed in regional myofascial pain
      b. Central—observed in fibromyalgia
    2. Source
      a. Neuropathic—not part of fibromyalgia; due to damaged or injured nerves, as in diabetes,
        trauma, and herinated disc
      b. Nociceptive—includes features of fibromyalgia (see Glossary for definitions)
        (i)   Hyperalgesia
        (ii) Neuroplasticity
        (iii) Causalgia
        (iv) Hyperpathia
      c. Non-nociceptive (allodynia)—can function as nociceptive fibers with chronic stimulation
        in fibromyalgia

Types of Wiring and Insulation: The Descending Tract

The brain sends signals back down the spinal cord via *adrenaline* (epinephrine) and *serotonin,* the principal neurotransmitters to the one million nerve fibers of the descending system. Serotonin is a remarkable chemical that we will talk more about later. In addition to nociception, serotonin is capable of regulating mood, arousal, aggression, sleep, learning, nerve growth, and appetite.

Finally, it's time to introduce a special subset of the peripheral nervous system, known as the *autonomic nervous system (ANS).* The ANS consists of two types of fibers, sympathetic and parasympathetic. The *sympathetic nervous system (SNS)* is our "fight or flight" mechanism. It releases adrenaline when we are threatened and "revs up the juices," resulting in aggressive behavior or self-protection. The ANS also regulates our pulse and blood pressure by constricting or dilating blood vessels. Additionally, the ANS can relax or contract muscles and regulates sweat, urine, and defecation reflexes. The ability of the SNS to stimulate sensory fibers that meld into the nociceptive pathway is extremely important. At the same time that nociceptive influences are being processed and sent up the spinothalamic tract, parallel signals from B (autonomic) fibers are received and sent to the limbic system of the brain via the *spinoreticular tract.* The limbic system helps modulate many of our emotions, including alertness, vigilance, and fear. Figure 4.2 illustrates normal nociceptive processes.

ORGANIC PAIN: LOCALIZED VERSUS CENTRAL PAIN; NOCICEPTIVE VERSUS NEUROPATHIC PAIN

Chronic pain can be *organic* (real) or *psychogenic,* when patients think their pain is physical. Organic sources of pain can be either *peripheral* or *central.*

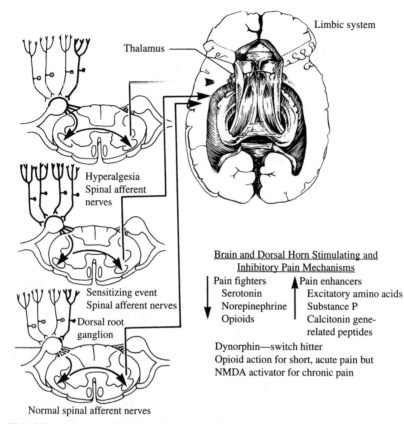

Brain and Dorsal Horn Stimulating and
Inhibitory Pain Mechanisms

Pain fighters	Pain enhancers
Serotonin	Excitatory amino acids
Norepinephrine	Substance P
Opioids	Calcitonin gene-related peptides

Dynorphin—switch hitter
Opioid action for short, acute pain but
NMDA activator for chronic pain

Fig. 4.2. *Pain amplification in fibromyalgia. Chronic sensitization of A-delta and C pain fibers leading to the thalamus and B fibers leading to the limbic system alters the normal system of releasing chemicals that enhance or fight pain.*

Peripheral pain results in muscular discomfort from local tender points. For instance, local injections of anesthetics such as novocaine or xylocaine can temporarily abolish pain at a specific site. Exercising a muscle can lead to pain in that muscle, as shown in Figure 4.3.

On the other hand, pain can emanate from brain and spinal cord pathways without any peripheral tissue or nociceptive input or stimulus. A classic example is something doctors call *phantom limb* pain. Let us say that a patient has had a leg amputated below the left knee but complains that the left ankle hurts. This seems impossible, but it happens all the time. This is due to a phenomenon known as *neuroplasticity,* where the brain has the adaptive capability to modify structure or function by growing nerve fibers, activating previously quiet nerves or creating hypersensitization.

Finally, chronic organic pain is either *nociceptive,* as in fibromyalgia, *non-nociceptive,* or *neuropathic.* Nociceptive pain occurs with chronic, repeated

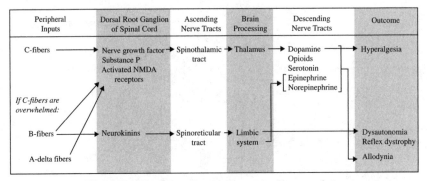

Fig. 4.3. *Chronic pain pathways in fibromyalgia.*

stimulation and can potentially produce tissue damage. In this circumstance, nonnociceptive fibers can act as nociceptive ones. Neuropathic pain results from a direct nerve injury that leads to nervous system dysfunction. Examples of neuropathic pain include diabetes, trauma, and herniated disc. These concepts are summarized in Table 4.1.

Hyperalgesia is an exaggerated response to a painful stimulus. Inappropriately increased hyperalgesia results when repeated stimuli from areas within tissues lower the thresholds for activating nociceptors. As a result, seemingly innocuous stimuli such as light touching can cause severe pain. For example, lack of oxygen to a capillary beneath the skin in the presence of a low pH (or acidic environment) is capable of activating, exciting, and sensitizing nociceptors. Another study has shown that fibromyalgia patients react to pain after stimulation with a carbon dioxide laser with greater nociceptive-evoked electrical activity than do healthy people. These actions lead to perceptual amplification, or a state of hypervigilance. *Hyperpathia* is an exaggerated response to a painful stimulus with continuing sensation of pain even after stimulation has ceased.

The mechanism or mechanisms that cause nociceptive pain loops to amplify pain rather than suppress pain in fibromyalgia is the subject of considerable scrutiny. A summary of what goes awry in fibromyalgia will now be reviewed.

MALADAPTIVE PAIN: WHAT CAUSES "PAIN WITHOUT PURPOSE"?

Maladaptive pain may be acute or chronic. One of the key features of maladaptive pain is increased sensitivity or hyper-responsiveness (allodynia or hyperalgesia). Pain perception is not hard-wired but changeable (termed plastic, or neuroplasticity). Small C fibers in the skin are easily activated by chemical, mechanical, or thermal energy. Even without noxious stimuli signals can arise spontaneously, which are converted into a neural impulse. Once sensitized by an inciting stimulus, various signals are sent through C-fiber nerves to the dorsal root ganglion of the spinal cord. If there are too many incoming signals, the spinal cord can have a hard time sorting them out and filtering them. The constant bombardment of noxious inputs by C-fibers leads to *central sensitization* (central refers to the spinal cord) and produces a *wind up* phenomenon. During the wind up process, pain is enhanced by each painful or nonpainful stimulus. Large A-delta fibers, which usually only transmit very noxious impulses, start carrying some of the signals usually carried by the C- fibers. Light touch is thus misinterpreted by the spinal cord and brain as hyperalgesia. Even the autonomic B fibers start carrying nociceptive stimuli to handle the overload. At this point, nonnociceptive fibers start to carry nociceptive signals. Known as allodynia, its maintenance becomes dependent upon continued central sensitization. In the dorsal root ganglion, increased discharges of second and third rung neurons in response to repetitive C-fiber stimulation takes place. This long-term hyperexcitability leads to a lower firing threshold and expansion of receptor fields, which are dependent upon size, location, and electrical thresholds for firing and selectivity of the receptor.

All this is accomplished through neurochemicals. Nociceptive signals cause the secretion of nerve growth factor, which produces a chemical known as substance P (for pain). Substance P facilitates nociception by altering spinal cord neurons (nerve cells) to incoming nociceptive peripheral signals. It migrates up and down the spinal cord, which ultimately leads to the generalization of fibromyalgia pain to other areas. Substance P turns on NMDA receptors. *NMDA receptors (N-methyl-D-aspartate)* are usually dormant and play no role in acute pain. Enhanced electrical depolarization causes calcium influx into nerve cells, which makes them more excitable. NMDA-related signals ascend to the brain and are processed in the thalamus (and B fibers in the limbic system).

The brain is now ready to meet this challenge by the inhibitory actions of neurotransmitters in the descending system. However, in fibromyalgia, serotonin levels are relatively low, which further causes more substance P to be made...this time in the brain. To clarify these complicated actions, we will now elaborate upon some of the chemicals we mentioned (and others) in more detail.

Important Chemical # 1: Substance P

Substance P stands for pain. Consisting of 11 amino acids (building blocks of protein), it is a neurotransmitter released in the dorsal root ganglion of the spinal cord, which results in greater pain perception by promoting blood vessel dilation and extravasation (leakage) into the plasma of a host of irritants, proinflammatory chemicals, and white blood cells (Fig. 4.3). Blood levels of substance P are normal in fibromyalgia, but four research centers have shown that its levels are increased in the spinal fluid of fibromyalgia patients. Sustained activation of substance P along with neurokinins lowers the pain threshold. Therefore, agents that block substance P may help patients with fibromyalgia. An example of this is capsaicin, a topical salve consisting of the chemical used in cayenne pepper and sold commercially as Zostrix or Dolorac. Nerve growth factor (chemical #5) is necessary for the production of substance P, and serotonin (chemical #2) inhibits it. Substance P stimulates the release of NMDA and neurokinin-1, which facilitate nociception.

Important Chemical # 2: Serotonin

Found in blood platelets, mast cells, the brain, and gastrointestinal cells, serotonin regulates the brain's ability to control pain and modulates mood, motivation, sleep, and behavior. Serotonin is also the major descending neurotransmitter of responses to nociception from the brain back to the spinal cord. Dr. Jon Russell at the University of Texas, San Antonio, has performed numerous studies suggesting that serotonin deficiency, both centrally and peripherally, is a key source of fibromyalgia pain and pathology. Serotonin is stored and released by platelets, cells that promote blood clotting. Normally, an amino acid known as *tryptophan* is metabolized to serotonin. For many years, L-tryptophan was available over the counter as a sleep aid. However, a contaminant in the manufacture of L-tryptophan produced a variant of the autoimmune disease scleroderma, and it was taken off the market in 1989. Unfortunately, in some patients, L-tryptophan travels via an alternate route, known as the *kynurenine pathway,* rather than via the serotonin pathway, which promotes anxiety and irritability. Russell's studies found that decreased serum levels of serotonin, tryptophan, and other amino acids in the spinal fluid in fibromyalgia suggest or lead to a variety of effects. These include less hypothalamic-pituitary-adrenal (or hormone-stress) axis activity (see Chapter 6), poor sleep, increased pain perception, alterations in substance P, and lower levels of growth and sex hormones.

Important Chemical # 3: Excitatory Amino Acids

Dr. Russell and others also found that a group of branched amino acids in addition to tryptophan are decreased in the spinal fluid of fibromyalgia patients. Stimulated, unmyelinated C fibers promote the release of these amino acids (e.g., valine, leucine, and isoleucine) and activate NMDA receptors, which produces painful signals (see Fig. 4.3). These receptors are usually inactivated, but become activated in sleep deprivation and chronic pain but not in acute pain. Fibromyalgia is perpetuated when neurokinin-1 and NMDA receptors remain activated and produce a sustained hyperexcitability state. An anesthetic known as *ketamine* selectively blocks NMDA receptors and produces the most dramatic fibromyalgia pain relief ever reported. Pain produced by NMDA receptors is only slightly blocked by opioids (morphine derivatives). Glutamate is a nociceptive stimulatory chemical mediator. Higher levels are associated with pain.

Important Chemical #4: Opiates and Endorphins

Enkephalins and endorphins are the body's natural opiates. These peptides (compounds with at least two amino acids) are parts of proteins. An *opiate* is a narcotic whose receptors play a role in chemical recognition and also have biologic actions. Endorphins are found in the skin and nerve cell membranes, and are biologically active neuropeptides. Their blood and spinal fluid levels are normal in fibromyalgia. In addition to producing euphoria via the sympathetic nervous system's connections to the limbic system, opiates can interact with serotonin to decrease pain perception. The administration of morphine near the spinal cord modestly decreases pain levels in fibromyalgia. *Tricyclic* antidepressants such as amitriptyline (Elavil), the drugs most commonly used to treat fibromyalgia, promote the release of endorphin, which may account for some of their efficacy. Another opioid, *dynorphin,* constricts blood vessels and also decreases acute pain but in chronic pain it becomes a "switch hitter," activating NMDA receptors and making chronic pain worse. We still know very little about this opiate.

Important Chemical #5: Nerve Growth Factor

According to Alice Larson at the University of Minnesota, spinal fluid levels of nerve growth factor are four times normal in fibromyalgia patients. Nerve growth factor dependent nociceptors account for 70% of all nociceptors. Essential for the survival of sensory and autonomic neurons during fetal development, nerve growth factor produces chemical and thermal (heat) hyperalgesia and stimulates the production of substance P in nerve endings.

Important Chemical #6: Nitric Oxide

Substance P and excitatory amino acids promote the release of nitric oxide. A potent blood vessel opener (dilator), agents that block nitric oxide also block NMDA receptors. Increased nitric oxide levels make one more hyperexcitable. It can increase muscle pain by decreasing the amount of ATP (energy packets) in muscle cells and cause muscle cells to die. Levels of nitric oxide in spinal fluid are increased in fibromyalgia.

Important Chemical #7: GABA

GABA, or gamma amino butyric acid, is an inhibitory neurotransmitter that acts at the dorsal horn and centrally, and whose concentrations are decreased in FM. Blocking spinal GABA results in allodynia by removing the inhibitors that control NMDA receptors. GABA promotes sleep and inhibits pain reflexes by blocking calcium channels and excitatory amino acids. Many of the drugs reviewed in chapter 22 promote GABA.

Important Chemical #8: Dopamine

Dopamine is a neurotransmitter that when activated has analgesic effects. Brain imaging demonstrates decreased dopamine responses in FM patients and dopaminergic agents generally have favorable effects upon periodic limb movement syndrome and other FM manifestations.

COMPLETING THE CAST OF CHARACTERS: OTHER IMPORTANT CHEMICALS

Other relevant chemicals are listed here for the sake of completeness. *Prostaglandins, bradykinins,* and *histamine* promote inflammation. *Neuropeptide Y* is a small breakdown product of norepinephrine that constricts blood vessels. Its levels are decreased in fibromyalgia and stress. *Acetylcholine, norepinephrine,* and *epinephrine* are also part of the autonomic nervous system and are reviewed in chapter 7. *Zinc* may inhibit pain and low *magnesium* levels amplify it as does *CGRP* (calcitonin gene-related peptide). *Cholecystokinin* is a neuropeptide with anti-opioid actions that may be important in treating functional bowel disease (see Chapter 13). *Somatostatin* (which blocks growth hormone) and angiotensin-2 also play bit roles in the nociceptive process. *C-fos* is a protein involved in the memory of pain.

ADDITIONAL FACTORS LEADING TO MALADAPTIVE PAIN

Are There Genetic Factors?

Research has indicated a strong familial component to the development of fibromyalgia. First-degree relatives of individuals with fibromyalgia display an eight-fold greater risk of developing fibromyalgia than those in the general population. These studies also show that family members of individuals with fibromyalgia are much more tender than the family members of controls, regardless of whether they have pain or not. Family members of fibromyalgia patients are also much more likely to have irritable bowel, headaches, and a host of other regional pain syndromes. This familial and personal co-aggregation of conditions which includes fibromyalgia was originally collectively termed *affective spectrum disorder,* and more recently *central sensitivity* syndrome, and chronic multisymptom illnesses. In population-based studies, the key symptoms that often co-aggregate besides pain are fatigue, memory difficulties, and mood disturbances. Twin studies suggest that approximately half of the risk of developing chronic widespread pain is due to genetic factors, and half is environmental.

Studies have begun to identify specific genetic polymorphisms that are associated with a higher risk of developing fibromyalgia. To date, the serotonin 5-HT2A receptor polymorphism T/T phenotype, beta-2 adrenergic receptor of the guanosine protein coupled stimulator receptor, serotonin transporter, dopamine 4 receptor, alpha-1 antitrypsin phenotype deficiency, and COMT (catecholamine *o*-methyl transferase) polymorphisms have all been noted to be seen in higher frequency in fibromyalgia. It is of note that all of the polymorphisms identified to date involve the metabolism or transport of monoamines, compounds that play a critical role in activity of the human stress response. It is likely that there are scores of genetic polymorphisms, involving other neuromodulators as well as monoamines, which in part determine an individuals' "set point" for pain and sensory processing.

Augmented Pain and Sensory Processing as a Hallmark of Fibromyalgia and Related Syndromes

Studies have found that fibromyalgia patients display low thresholds to stimuli, and the correlation between the results of auditory and pressure pain threshold testing suggested that some of this was due to shared variance, and some unique to one stimulus or the other. The notion that fibromyalgia and related syndromes might represent biological amplification of all sensory stimuli has significant support from functional imaging studies that suggest that the insula is the most consistently hyperactive region (see below). This region has been noted to play a critical role in sensory integration, with the posterior insula serving a purer sensory role, and the anterior insula being associated with the emotional processing of sensations.

Specific Mechanisms That May Lead to a Low Pain Threshold in Fibromyalgia

There are two different specific pathogenic mechanisms in fibromyalgia that have been identified using experimental pain testing: 1) an absence of descending analgesic activity, and 2) increased wind-up or temporal summation. *Simplistically stated, FM patients fail to suppress pain and with repetitive pain signals amplify pain.* Much of the work detailed below comes from Dr. Roland Staud and his colleagues at the University of Florida.

Attenuated DNIC in fibromyalgia. In healthy humans and laboratory animals, application of an intense painful stimulus for two to five minutes produces generalized whole-body analgesia. This analgesic effect, termed "diffuse noxious inhibitory controls" (DNIC), has been consistently observed to be attenuated or absent in groups of FM patients, compared to healthy controls. The DNIC response in humans is believed to be partly mediated by descending opioidergic pathways and in part by descending serotonergic-noradrenergic pathways. In fibromyalgia, the accumulating data suggests that opioidergic activity is normal or even increased, in that levels of cerebrospinal fluid (CSF) enkephalins are roughly twice as high in FM and idiopathic low back pain patients as in healthy controls. Moreover, PET data show that baseline mu-opioid receptor binding is decreased in multiple pain processing regions in the brains of FM patients, consistent (but not pathognomonic) with the hypothesis that there is increased release of endogenous mu-opioid ligands in FM leading to high baseline occupancy of the receptors. The biochemical and imaging findings suggesting increased activity of endogenous opioidergic systems in FM are consistent with the anecdotal experience that opioids are generally ineffective analgesics in patients with FM and related conditions. In contrast, studies have shown the opposite for serotonergic and noradrenergic activity in FM. Studies have shown that the principal metabolite of norepinephrine, 3-methoxy-4-hydroxyphenethylene (MPHG), is lower in the CSF of FM patients, and nearly any type of compound that simultaneously raises both serotonin and norepinephrine (tricyclics, duloxetine, milnacipran, tramadol) has been shown to be efficacious in treating FM and related conditions.

Increased wind-up in fibromyalgia. Experimental pain testing studies have also suggested that some individuals with fibromyalgia may have evidence of wind-up, indicative of evidence of central sensitization (not to be confused with central *sensitivity*, which is a more general phenomenon). In animal models, that finding is associated with excitatory amino acid (e.g., glutamate) and Substance P hyperactivity. Several independent studies have shown that patients with FM have approximately threefold higher concentrations of Substance P in CSF, when compared with normal controls. Another important neurotransmitter in pain processing, and one that likely is playing some role in FM, is glutamate. Glutamate (Glu) is a major excitatory neurotransmitter within the central nervous system, and cerebrospinal fluid levels of glutamate are twice as high in FM patients than controls. Not only are these levels elevated, but a recent study using proton spectroscopy demonstrated that the glutamate levels in the insula in fibromyalgia changes in response to changes in both clinical and experimental pain when patients are treated with acupuncture. Furthermore, medications that seem to act by reducing the release of these excitatory neurotransmitters (e.g., pregabalin, gabapentin) ameliorate fibromyalgia.

Thus, a number of lines of evidence point to the fact that fibromyalgia is a state of heightened pain or sensory processing, and that this might occur because of high levels of neurotransmitters that increase pain transmission, and/or low levels of neurotransmitters that decrease pain transmission (see Figure 17.1).

Abnormalities on Functional Neuroimaging

Functional neural imaging enables investigators to visualize how the brain processes the sensory experience of pain. The primary modes of functional imaging that have been used in FM include functional Magnetic Resonance Imaging (fMRI), Single Photon Emission Computed Tomography (SPECT), and Positron Emission Tomography (PET), and proton spectroscopy (H-MRS).

Single-Photon-Emission Computed Tomographic (SPECT) was the first functional neuroimaging technique to be used in fibromyalgia. Initial data has indicated that both the caudate and the thalamus of FM patients had decreased blood flow. More detailed studies found hyperperfusion in FM patients within the somatosensory cortex and hypoperfusion in the anterior and posterior cingulate, the amygdala, medial frontal and parahippocampal gyrus, and the cerebellum. One longitudinal treatment trial used SPECT imaging to assess changes in rCBF following administration of amitriptyline within 14 FM patients. After three months of treatment with amitriptyline, increases in rCBF in the bilateral thalamus and the basal ganglia were observed. Since the same two regions had been implicated previously, these data suggest that amitriptyline may normalize the altered blood flow, thereby reducing pain symptoms.

Functional MRI (fMRI). fMRI is a non-invasive brain imaging technique that relies on changes in the relative concentration of oxygenated to deoxygenated hemoglobin within the brain. Regions of increased activity included the primary and secondary somatosensory cortex, the insula, and the anterior cingulate, all regions commonly observed in fMRI studies of healthy normal subjects during painful stimuli. Interestingly, when pain-free controls were subjected to pressures that evoked equivalent pain ratings in the fibromyalgia patients, similar activation patterns were observed. These findings were entirely consistent with the "left-shift" in stimulus-response function noted with experimental pain testing, and suggest that fibromyalgia patients experience an increased gain or "volume setting" in brain sensory processing systems. These data are consistent with a plethora of evidence in the pain field that there are different regions of the brain responsible for pain processing devoted to sensory intensity versus affective aspects of pain sensation, and suggest that the former and latter are largely independent of each other. The presence of catastrophizing, a patient's negative or pessimistic appraisal of their pain, influences both the sensory and affective dimensions of pain on fMRI in fibromyalgia.

PET has been used in several studies in fibromyalgia. Preliminary work suggests that PET attenuates dopaminergic activity and may be playing a role in pain transmission in fibromyalgia, and there is also evidence of decreased *mu* opiod receptor availability (possibly due to increased release of endogenous *mu* opioids) in fibromyalgia.

Behavioral and Psychological Factors

In addition to neurobiological mechanisms, behavioral and psychological factors also play a role in symptom expression in many FM patients. The rate of current psychiatric co-morbidity in patients with FM may be as high as 30 to 60% in tertiary care settings, and the rate of lifetime psychiatric disorders even higher. Depression and anxiety disorders are the most commonly seen. However, these rates may be artifactually elevated by virtue of the fact that most of these studies have been performed in tertiary care centers. Individuals who meet ACR criteria for FM who are identified in the general population do not have nearly this high a rate of identifiable psychiatric conditions.

SUMMING UP

Fibromyalgia is characterized by abnormalities in the central nervous system's processing of sensory input of pain signals. Patients with fibromyalgia hurt when and where they should not. Pain amplification could be the result of the release of neurotransmitters where the sustained release of certain chemicals results in more pain. Some of the possible disruptions in pain circuitry have been reviewed, but we still know relatively little about what really goes on.

FOR FURTHER READING

Abeles AM, Pillinger MH, Solitar BM, Abeles M. Narrative review: The pathophysiology of fibromyalgia. 2007; *146*: 726–734.

Arnold LM, Hudson JI, Hess EV, *et al.* Family study of fibromyalgia. *Arthritis Rheum* 2005; *50*: 944–952.

Bendsten L, Norregasard, Jensen R, Ollesen J. Evidence of qualitatively altered nociception in patients with fibromyalgia. *Arthritis Rheum 40*, 1997: 98–102.

Buskila D. Genetics of chronic pain states. *Best Prac Res Clin Rheumatol* 2007; *21*: 535–547.

Gracely RH, Petzke F, Wolf JM, Clauw DJ. Functional magnetic resonance imaging evidence of augmented pain processing in fibromyalgia, *Arthritis Rheum* 2002; *52*: 1577–1584.

Harris RE, Clauw DJ, Scott DJ, *et al.* Decreased central mu-opioid receptor availability in fibromyalgia. *J Neurosci* 2007; *27*: 10,000–10,006.

Millan MJ, The induction of pain: an integrative review. *Prog Neurobiol* 1999, 1–164.

Price DD, Staud R, Robinson ME, *et al.* Enhanced temporal summation of second pain and its central modulation in fibromyalgia patients. *Pain* 2002; *99*: 49–59.

Smith SB, Maxiner DW, Fillingim RB, *et al.* Large candidate gene association study reveals genetic risk factors and therapeutic targets for fibromyalgia. *Arthritis Rheum* 2012; *64*: 584–593.

Vaeroy H, Helle R, Forre O, *et al.* Elevated CSF levels of substance P and high incidence of Raynaud's phenomenon in patients with fibromyalgia syndrome. *Pain 32*, 1988: 21–26.

5
What's Wrong with My Muscles?

The human body...indeed is like a ship; its bones being the stiff standing-rigging, and the sinews the small running ropes, that manage all the motions.

Herman Melville (1819–1891)

Since most fibromyalgia patients complain of aching and spasm in their muscles, common sense suggests that there must be something wrong with the muscle. This is easier said than agreed upon. For the last 80 years, researchers have been looking for the key to muscle pathology in fibromyalgia. As of this writing, there are highly respected investigators who feel that there is little if anything wrong with fibromyalgia muscles. However, other equally regarded researchers have presented evidence that abnormal muscle metabolism is nevertheless important for what goes awry in the disorder.

Why are there such discrepancies? Let's explore what goes on in our muscles.

IS THERE ANYTHING WRONG WITH MUSCLE
STRUCTURE IN FIBROMYALGIA?

Our body has 640 different muscles, which constitute as much as 40% of our weight. When physicians look at muscles of fibromyalgia patients under a simple microscope, they generally appear normal. In fact, muscles must be looked at under an electron microscope (which magnifies the tissue thousands of times) in order to find any consistent abnormalities. In this setting there are subtle alterations, including the deposition of a chemical, glycogen, swollen and abnormal cell organelles known as mitochondria, increased DNA fragmentation ragged red fibers, and smeared muscle cell membranes. Some investigators have shown that magnesium levels are low in the muscles of fibromyalgia patients. So where are the disagreements? Fibromyalgia patients are generally deconditioned. In other words, they are out of shape. Of course, many more people are out of shape than have fibromyalgia, but studies of muscles from out-of-shape people also show some of these alterations.

WHAT ABOUT MUSCLE FUNCTION?

If fibromyalgia muscles don't look very different from normal muscles under the microscope, where else can we look for muscle pathology? Muscle strength can be decreased or normal in fibromyalgia, and published studies conflict as to whether or not muscle fatigue is present. Nevertheless, people who are out of shape also have decreased muscle strength.

Let's look at blood flow to muscles. Muscles are fueled by oxygen, which is supplied and carried by arteries. Some muscles in fibromyalgia do not get enough oxygen. "Angina" of the muscles can develop, producing pain if the oxygen supply is decreased. (The heart is a muscle. Angina is cardiac chest pain brought on when not enough blood is supplied to the heart muscle via the coronary arteries.) Individuals who don't exercise regularly also have low tissue oxygenation. However, out-of-shape people don't necessarily have all the features reported in the *microcirculation* (small arteries and capillaries) of fibromyalgia patients. The diminished oxygen supply may also have to do with interactions between the ANS and the muscle in fibromyalgia. Other investigators minimize the role of the ANS and have performed experiments suggesting that the shape of red blood cell membranes is altered in fibromyalgia or the capillary coverings are thicker. This could adversely influence blood flow in small capillaries and prevent oxygen from reaching muscles and other tissues. A consequence of this is the release of chemicals including histamine, prostaglandin, and bradykinin, which can further sensitize afferent nerve endings.

The body's immediate energy fuel is adenosine triphosphate (ATP). An enzyme involved in the production of ATP in muscles may be defective in fibromyalgia. Muscles become slower to consume glucose to produce energy, which diminishes energy reserves. When this happens, fibromyalgia patients don't utilize enough oxygen to meet their energy needs. Additionally, several researchers have examined the biochemistry of muscles by using a magnetic spectroscope not too different from the technology used in magnetic resonance imaging (MRI) scanning. A spectroscope is an instrument that analyzes light waves emitted by tissues. Some investigators report that fibromyalgia muscles have lower than normal levels of high-energy phosphates, but others counter that this condition is also seen in deconditioning.

Electrical activity in muscles can be assessed by an electromyogram (EMG). This "cardiogram of the muscles" also is normal when performed conventionally. However, if the EMG is performed with special maneuvers not usually performed with standard testing, fibromyalgic muscles may have difficulty relaxing after exertion and, when they are deprived of oxygen, have more spontaneous electrical activity.

MICROTRAUMA AND "TAUT BANDS" ARE PROBABLY RESPONSIBLE FOR MOST OF WHAT GOES WRONG WITH MUSCLES IN FIBROMYALGIA

Among others, Soren Jacobsen in Sweden and Robert Bennett at the University of Oregon put together concepts that might best explain what occurs in fibromyalgic muscles, developing what is known as the *microtrauma* or *taut band* hypothesis. Although unproven, it makes a lot of sense and represents a reasonable explanation worthy of the reader's time and effort to understand.

When healthy but sedentary people exert themselves abnormally, such as on a ski or hiking trip, this unaccustomed exertion results in muscle soreness and stiffness. Some of this pain could be due to microscopic muscle tears resulting in leakage of chemicals that produce discomfort. This usually lasts a day or two, and then the body's repair mechanisms take care of the problem. In fibromyalgia, the soreness and stiffness become chronic. How does this happen? Follow the sequences illustrated in Figure 5.1 as we describe this hypothesis.

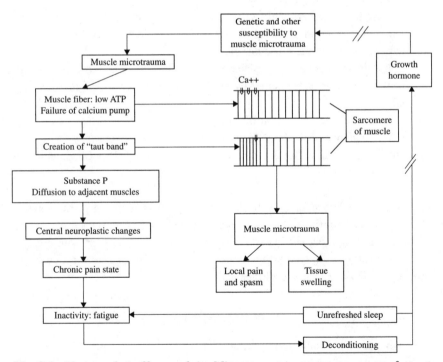

Fig. 5.1. *The muscle in fibromyalgia. Microtrauma creates a sequence of events leading to muscle spasm and not enough oxygen getting to muscles, which produces pain.*

When a focal injury affects a muscle fiber, it contains both relaxed and contracted units, or sarcomeres. This causes potassium to leave muscles and sarcomeres to stimulate Type C unmyelinated pain nerve endings. The ensuing hyperexcitability of spinal cord neurons sensitizes second-order neurons. Nonnociceptive impulses produce allodynia, and nociceptive impulses hyperalgesia. In turn, a calcium-ATP (or energy) pump is activated, unleashing events that produce a *taut band* (Figure 5.1). In other words, some of the muscle becomes as tight as a rubber band, while adjacent muscle relaxes. As a result of this chain of events, insufficient oxygen reaches muscles. Additionally, there are focal decreases in critical muscle enzyme levels that provide energy and fuel, as well as the release of substance P to nearby sarcomeres, producing pain and spasm. Some of these chemicals sensitize the nervous system, which perpetuates the vicious cycle of pain and spasm. In the last decade, additional insights into the pathophysiology of the role of muscles in fibromyalgia have been published:

a. It is probable that muscle fatigue in fibromyalgia comes from the brain more than from muscles
b. Muscle fiber velocity is higher in fibromyalgia on electromyography
c. Dopamine, norepinephrine and serotonin (biogenic amines) are depleted in patients with chronic muscular pain
d. There is more anaerobic metabolism in fibromyalgia muscles than in healthy controls as measured by lactic acid which makes the muscles less effective
e. Calcium channel activation of surface signals/receptors (kinases) on cells in the thalamus of the brain is associated with chronic muscle pain.
f. Diffuse noxious inhibitory controls (DNIC) discussed in Chapter 4 also occurs in muscles

Also, growth hormone and its liver by-product, insulin-like growth factor 1 (IGF-1), are made during deep sleep and promote repair of muscles damaged by microtrauma. When patients sleep poorly, this repair is interfered with. Tender points occur at muscle-tendon junctions, where mechanical forces produce the most injury. This is discussed further in the next chapter.

SUMMING UP

Although muscles usually look normal in fibromyalgia, and although many of the changes described in muscle tissues reflect being out of shape, there are probably certain unique self-perpetuating events that produce muscle pain and spasm through the interplay of microtrauma, pain, chemicals, and unrefreshing sleep. Muscle pain is evoked by nociceptors stimulated by ATP and a low tissue pH. Excitation of muscle nociceptors leads to central sensitization.

FOR FURTHER READING

Mense S. Muscle Pain: Mechanisms and Clinical Significance. *Deutsches Artzeblatt International*, 2008; *105*: 214–219.

Norregaard J. Muscle function, psychometric scoring and prognosis in patients with widespread pain and tenderness (fibromyalgia). *Danish Med Bulletin 45*, 1998: 256–267.

Olsen NJ, Park JH. Skeletal muscle abnormalities in patients with fibromyalgia *Amer J Med Sci 315*, 1998: 351–358.

Shang Y, Gurley K, Symons B, *et al.* Noninvasive of characterization of muscle blood flow, oxygenation, and metabolism in women with fibromyalgia. *Arthritis Res Ther* 2012; *14*: R236.

Staud R. Peripheral pain mechanisms in chronic widespread pain. *Best Prac Res Clin Rheumatol* 2011; 25: 155–164.

6

How Do Stress, Sleep, Hormones, and the Immune System Interact and Relate to Fibromyalgia?

Canst thou not minister to a mind diseased/Pluck from the memory a rooted sorrow/Raze out the written troubles of the brain/And with some sweet oblivious antidote/Cleanse the stuffed bosom of that perilous stuff/ Which weighs upon the heart?

William Shakespeare (1564–1616), *Macbeth*, 5:3-40

In medical school, students learn about the human body by *organ system.* They spend a few weeks on the heart, then the lung, followed by the gastrointestinal tract. Eventually the whole body is covered. One of the fascinating developments in the last decade has been the functional linkage and new connections of seemingly diverse body systems. Fibromyalgia research finally hit its stride when important studies connected the nervous system, the endocrine (hormone) system, and the immune system. This enabled physicians to devise improved strategies to help fibromyalgia patients. Basic background information provided in this chapter will be expanded upon in later parts of the book when we review treatments.

THE "STRESS HORMONE," OR HYPOTHALAMIC-PITUITARY-ADRENAL AXIS

Within the brain is a small region known as the *hypothalamus.* It makes releasing hormones that travel down a short path to the pituitary gland, which makes stimulating hormones. The stimulating hormones send signals to tissues where hormones are manufactured for specialized functions. Table 6.1 and Figure 6.1 show how thyroid, cortisol, insulin, breast milk, and growth hormone are made along the hypothalamic-pituitary axis and the hypothalamic-pituitary-adrenal (HPA) axis.

Table 6.1. *Important Hormones Derived from the Hypothalamic-Pituitary Axis*

Hypothalamus (Releasers)	Pituitary (Stimulators)	Peripheral tissues (Hormones)
Corticotropin-releasing hormone	Adrenocorticotropic hormone	Cortisone
Thyrotropin-releasing hormone	Thyroid-stimulating hormone	Thyroid
Growth hormone-releasing hormone	Growth hormone	
Prolactin-releasing factor	Prolactin	Breast milk
Gonadotropin-releasing hormone	Follicle-stimulating hormone, luteinizing hormone	Estrogen, progesterone

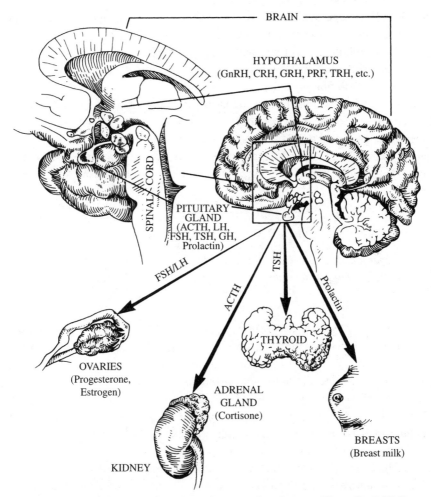

Fig. 6.1. *Hypothalamic and pituitary hormonal pathways. (From D. J. Wallace, The Lupus Book. New York: Oxford University Press, 1995, p. 123; reprinted with permission.)*

STRESS AND THE HPA AXIS

We have already mentioned that emotional stress can bring on or aggravate fibromyalgia. At the National Institutes of Health and the University of Michigan, studies have firmly established some of the factors important in this relationship. The role of corticotropin-releasing hormone (CRH), the precursor or ancestor of the steroid known as *cortisol,* has been the focus of much of this work. Even though CRH levels are normal in fibromyalgia, CRH responses (stress responses) to different forms of stimulation are blunted. CRH has many important interactions other than leading to the production of steroids. Its expression can be increased by stress, serotonin, and estrogen. Endorphins promote the secretion of CRH. Decreased sympathetic nervous system activity in the adrenal glands and substance P, as well as nitric oxide, can turn off CRH production. Cortisol levels vary with the time of day, and its secretion is lowest in the middle of the night. Rats with abnormally low stress responses develop many of the features we associate with fibromyalgia.

How do these interrelationships translate into a fibromyalgia patient's feeling of being unwell? The answer is not clear. However, these studies suggest that fibromyalgia patients do not respond normally to acute stress and do not release enough adrenalin. This leads to a chronic stress state to which the body reacts by making things worse, creating a vicious cycle that perpetuates the unwell feeling.

SLEEP AND FIBROMYALGIA

The average, healthy, well-adjusted adult gets up at seven-thirty in the morning feeling just terrible.

Jean Kerr (1923–2003)

Between 2 and 15% of any given population and 60 and 90% of FM patients have nonrestorative sleep, or waking up feeling not refreshed. First reported with FM in the 1970s by Moldofsky's group in Toronto, alpha wave intrusion into delta wave sleep is noted on polysomnograms (an electrical tracing of the brain while sleeping, or sort of a cardiogram of the brain) during stages 2–4 of non-rapid eye movement (non-REM) sleep. Other findings noted include increase in stage I sleep, reduction in delta sleep, and an increase in the number of arousals. This leads to one being in bed for eight hours or so, but waking up not feeling rested. Moldofsky's group has identified three distinct patterns of alpha sleep activity in FM: phasic alpha-delta activity (50%), tonic alpha continuous throughout non-REM sleep (20%), and low alpha in the remaining 30%. The phasic group had the greatest number of symptoms and lowest sleep time. Increased fragmented sleep has been documented additionally by greater numbers of arousals and alpha-K complexes (which promotes arousal, fatigue, and muscular symptoms) in the syndrome. Electrocardiograms demonstrate increased sympathetic nervous system activity overnight, while healthy individuals report a decline with sleep. FM and pain have been associated with a higher proportion of stage I non-REM sleep, fewer sleep spindles, and less sleep spindle frequency activity (usually seen in Phase 2 sleep), suggesting that the mechanism relates to thalamocortical mechanisms of spindle generation. Cyclic altering patterns during sleep, which express instability of the level of vigilance that manifests the brain's fatigue in preserving and regulating the macrostructure of sleep is more often present in FM. See Figure 6.2.

Nonrestorative sleep is felt to derive from decreases in growth in growth hormone secretion as measured by IGF-1 (insulin-like growth hormone). We have 640 muscles in our body which undergo microtrauma during our daytime activities. Once asleep, growth hormone and melatonin secretion is increased which heals the microtrauma experienced by our muscles. In other words, abnormal electrical activity interferes with a sound sleep. These changes are more pronounced with menstruation, stress, pain, trauma, infection, urinating at night, and barometric changes. Forced awakenings (fragmented sleep) leads to the loss of DNIC and is associated with increased achiness.

Ten to thirty percent of FM patients exhibit another pattern of sleep pathology which can be documented via a sleep study: *restless legs syndrome*, also known as *sleep myoclonus* or *periodic limb movement syndrome*. These patients experience an alpha wave burst followed by limb movement, and may have excess sympathetic tone, more movement arousals, less stage 3 and 4 sleep. They do not respond to usual sleep aids, and report that their legs shoot

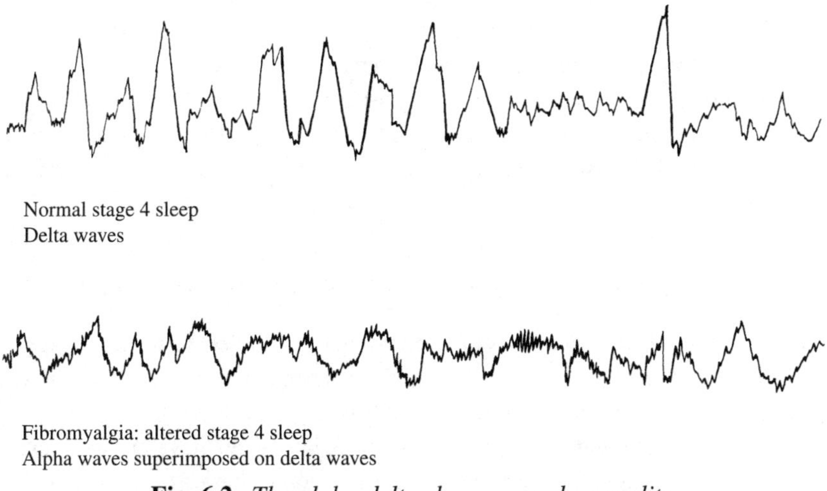

Normal stage 4 sleep
Delta waves

Fibromyalgia: altered stage 4 sleep
Alpha waves superimposed on delta waves

Fig. 6.2. *The alpha-delta sleep wave abnormality.*

out, lift, jerk, or go into spasm. Bed partners are often the first to alert one that this is present.

Respiratory flow dynamics during sleep in FM have been surveyed. While initial reports suggested that it may correlate with an increased numbers with sleep apnea (especially in men) its true prevalence is only 5%. It is probable that upper-airway resistance syndrome (UARS) rather than sleep apnea or hypopnea is present in the overwhelming majority of FM patients.

HORMONES AND SLEEP

"...the innocent sleep. Sleep that knits up the ravell'd sleeve of care. The each day's life, sore labor's bath. Balm of hurt minds, great nature's second course. Chief nourisher of life's feast.

Shakespeare's *Macbeth*

Even fully-grown adults require growth hormone for a variety of purposes. Most growth hormone is produced when we are in slow (delta) wave sleep. Levels of a product of growth hormone known as IGF-1 (*insulin-like growth factor, also called somatomedin C*) are decreased by 30% in fibromyalgia, especially in the early morning. CRH also promotes the release of a chemical that blocks growth hormone secretion. Dr. Robert Bennett has theorized that the low levels of growth hormone observed in fibromyalgia patients (as measured by their by-products, IGF-1) make them more susceptible to muscle trauma because micro-trauma occurring during the day cannot be repaired at night. Patients with low growth hormone levels have decreased energy, exercise capacity, muscle weakness, and impaired cognition.

What does this mean in a practical sense? Abnormal electrical waves keep fibromyalgia patients up at night, which, in turn, prevents enough growth hormone from being made to repair and restore their muscles. Also, sleep can be augmented by the production of chemicals such as interleukin-1, tumor necrosis factor-alpha, acetylcholine, nitric oxide, and a hormone made by another part of the brain (pineal gland) known as *melatonin.* Moreover, fragmentation of sleep occurs with menstruation, stress, pain, trauma, infection, or a change in the weather.

THE ROLE OF OTHER HORMONES IN FIBROMYALGIA

Additional hormones have been superficially studied in fibromyalgia. *Dehydroepiandrosterone (DHEA),* an adrenal hormone, may be decreased in the syndrome. The *thyroid* hormone level is normal, but its responses to hypothalamic stimuli are blunted. A subset of fibromyalgia patients have elevated levels of *prolactin,* a hormone responsible for the secretion of breast milk, which may affect the immune system and muscles.

THE FINAL LINKAGE: CONNECTING HORMONES AND
NERVES WITH THE IMMUNE SYSTEM AND CYTOKINES

What goes wrong with the immune system in fibromyalgia? When the body is attacked, the immune system comes to the rescue. We have a very sophisticated immune surveillance system, and it may come as a surprise that this system is reasonably intact in fibromyalgia. For example, in fibromyalgia studies of immune responsiveness, T-cell and B-cell counts, levels of autoantibodies (such as antinuclear antibody and rheumatoid factor), and the effectiveness of immunizations and allergy shots are usually normal. When I explain this to some patients, they ask why they develop so many infections or have lupus-like signs such as Raynaud's phenomenon (in which the fingers turn different colors in cold weather). There are explanations for this, some related to the ANS (see the next chapter) and others related to overlapping features with chronic fatigue syndrome (see Chapter 13).

One of the immune system's components involves a group of cellular protein hormones known as *cytokines*. Cytokines play a role in the growth and development of T and B cells and have exotic names such as *interleukins* and *interferons*. They amplify or "gear up" T cells and B cells, which are types of white blood cells known as *lymphocytes*. Even though cytokine blood levels are normal in patients with fibromyalgia, the administration of cytokines to treat diseases (such as alpha-interferon to manage hepatitis or interleukin-2 for advanced cancer) *induces* or causes fibromyalgia. Table 6.2 lists how cytokines can influence manifestations of fibromyalgia. As the first doctor to document this in the medical literature, I was amazed when my patients with advanced cancer at the City of Hope Medical Center developed fatigue, muscle aches, and difficulty connecting their thoughts within days of receiving interleukin-2. These fibromyalgia-like symptoms lasted for several weeks and then disappeared even if no further therapy was given.

Hormones and cytokines play an important role in the disturbances reported in FM. Behavioral makeup, stress, estrogen release and sympathetic nerve activity, and interleukin-1 beta (IL-1 beta) all lead to the release of CRH (corticotropin releasing hormone) which indirectly blocks growth hormone secretion. IL-1 independently promotes fatigue, sleep, muscle aches and blocks the release of substance P. Chronic insomnia is associated with a shift of IL-6 and tumor necrosis factor secretion from the nighttime to daytime as well as hypersecretion of cortisol. This leads to daytime fatigue and difficulty sleeping. See Figure 6.3.

How does this relate to fibromyalgia? Increased IL-8 function has been consistently demonstrated in multiple studies by different groups, including ours. Moreover, IL-8 has been shown to correlate with symptoms and not to be associated with depressed FM. IL-8 levels are closely tied to autonomic function and the findings of these increased levels could be due to the dysautonomia seen in fibromyalgia and related conditions. Abnormalities in IL-6 and IL-1 receptor

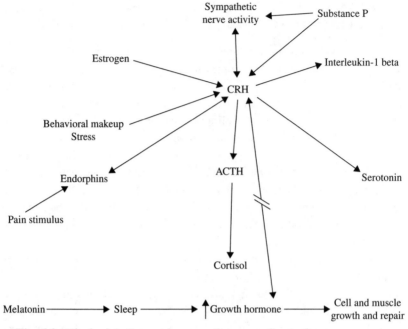

Fig. 6.3. *The body's "stress hormone" system. Cortisol, estrogen, pain, chemicals, muscles, sleep, stress, and the ANS all interact with each other.*

antagonist activity have also been shown (Table 6.2). One of the problems in evaluating cytokines is that measuring blood levels are not helpful. Part of this is because cytokines don't cross the blood-brain barrier very well. It turns out that a cell type in the brain known as the *glial cell* can make pro-inflammatory cytokines and signal pain activation, but are not measurable in the blood. Exciting ongoing studies will inform us about pain in fibromyalgia in the next few years.

What about Autoantibodies?

Anti-serotonin antibody, anti-ganglioside antibody, and anti-phospholipid antibody have been shown to be different in patients and controls, but the

Table 6.2. *How Cytokines Can Influence Fibromyalgia*

Cytokine	Association
IL-1 beta	hyperalgesia, fatigue, sleep, muscle aches, blocks substance P
IL-2	muscle aches, cognitive dysfunction
IL-6	fatigue, hyperalgesia, depression, activates sympathetic nervous system
IL-8	production stimulated by substance P, mediates sympathetic nervous system pain
IL-10	blocks pain
TNF-alpha	produces sleep, allodynia, increases NMDA activity, regulates substance P expression

applicability of these findings is not yet clear. Anti-thromboplastin antibody, anti-polymer antibody, anti-68/84, and anti-45kDa have been each evaluated in one cross-sectional study and have shown increased levels in FM. Reviews of the literature suggest that antinuclear antibody, anti-thyroid antibodies, anti-silicone antibodies, anti glutamic acid decarboxylase are not informative in FM.

This inconsistent increase in antibodies to a number of antigens may be a non-specific finding that arises from a subtle shift in immune function in this spectrum of illness. In the closely related chronic fatigue syndrome and Gulf War Illnesses, investigators have noted a shift from a TH1 to TH2 (immune reactive to immune suppressive) immune response, which would be expected to lead to increased production of non-specific antibodies.

Our group and others has found increased IL-6, IL-8 and IL-1 receptor antagonist activity in fibromyalgia patients. Cytokine production is decreased in FM patients who are chronically stressed.

Figure 6.3 illustrates some of the disease interrelationships of hormones, sleep, and the immune system.

SUMMING UP

Certain hormone levels (especially CRH) are normal in fibromyalgia but respond sluggishly, especially to stress. Abnormal electrical brain waves interrupt normal sleep patterns, and this may influence normal responses of growth hormone, which, in turn, affects muscles. Administering cytokines can cause or improve fibromyalgia, and these chemicals are interconnected with hormonal and pain pathways.

We now are ready to add another piece of this puzzle to what has already been introduced. Let's welcome the autonomic nervous system.

FOR FURTHER READING

Behm FG, Gavin IM, Karpenko O, *et al.* Unique immunologic patterns in fibromyalgia. *BMC Clin Pathol* 2012; *12*: 25.

Crofford LJ. The hypothalamus-pituitary-adrenal axis in the fibromyalgia syndrome. *J Musculoskeletal Pain 4*, 1996: 181–200.

Hening WA, Caivano CK. Restless legs syndrome: A common disorder in patients with rheumatologic conditions. *Seminars Arthritis Rheum* 2008; *38*: 55–62.

Herrmann M, Scholmerich J, Straub RH. Stress and rheumatic diseases. *Rheum Dis Clin North America 26*, 2000: 737–764.

Moldofsky H. The chronobiologic theory of fibromyalgia. *J Musculoskeletal Pain 1*, 1996: 49–59.

Moldofsky H. The significance of the sleeping-waking brain for the understanding of widespread musculoskeletal pain and fatigue in fibromyalgia syndrome and allied conditions. *Joint Bone Spine* 2008; *75*: 397–402.

Pillemer SR, Bradley LA, Crofford LJ., Moldofsky H, Chrousos GP. The neuroscience and endocrinology of fibromyalgia. *Arthritis Rheum 40*, 1997: 1928–1929.

Russell IJ, Vaeroy H, Javors, *et al*. Cerebrospinal fluid biogenic amine metabolites in fibromyalgia/fibrositis syndrome and rheumatoid arthritis. *Arthritis Rheum 35*, 1992: 550–556.

Uceyler N, Hauser W, Sommer C. Systemic review with meta-analysis: cytokines in fibromyalgia syndrome. *BMC Musculoskel Dis* 2011; *12*: 245.

Wallace DJ, Linker-Israeli M, Hallegua D, *et al*. Cytokines play an aetiopathogenetic role in fibromyalgia: a hypothesis and pilot study. *Rheumatology* 2001; *40*: 743–749.

7

What Is the Autonomic Nervous System?

Absence of psychoneurotic illness may be health but it is not life.
                                                              D.W. Winnicott,
                                                        Playing and Reality, 1971

The autonomic nervous system (ANS) has already been introduced; let's summarize what we know about it so far. Part of the peripheral nervous system, the ANS consists of the *sympathetic nervous system (SNS),* which consists of outflow from the thoracic and upper lumbar spine, and the *parasympathetic nervous system* (PNS), including outflow from the cranial nerves emanating from the upper spine and also from the mid-lumbar to the sacral areas at the buttock region. Several neurochemicals help transmit autonomic instructions. These include *epinephrine* (adrenaline), *norepinephrine* (noradrenalin), *dopamine,* and *acetylcholine.* This chapter will focus on how abnormalities in the regulation of the ANS cause many of the symptoms and signs observed in fibromyalgia.

THE WORKINGS OF THE ANS

Our body has numerous receptors or surveillance sensors that detect heat, cold, and inflammation. These ANS sensors perform a function known as *autoregulation.* As an example of how the ANS normally works, why don't we pass out when we suddenly jump out of bed? Because the ANS instantly constricts our blood vessels peripherally and dilates them centrally. In other words, as blood is pooled to the heart and the brain, the ANS adjusts our blood pressure and regulates our pulse, or heart rate, so that we don't collapse. On the local level, these sensors dilate or constrict flow from blood vessels. They can secondarily contract and relax muscles, open and close lung airways, or cause us to sweat. For instance, ANS sensors can tone muscles, regulate urine, and regulate bowel movements, as well as dilate or constrict our pupils. The SNS arm of the ANS is our "fight or flight" system, releasing epinephrine and norepinephrine as well as a neurochemical called *dopamine.* Whereas the SNS often acts as an acute stress response, the PNS arm tends to protect and conserve body processes and resources. The SNS and PNS sometimes work at cross purposes, but frequently

Table 7.1. *Normal Autonomic Functions*

Area	Sympathetic nervous system	Parasympathetic nervous system
Neurotransmitter	Norepinephrine, epinephrine Acetylcholine, dopamine	Acetylcholine
Saliva	Increases	Increases
Tears	Decreases	Increases
Pupils	Dilates	Constricts
Heart	Increases contraction, blood pressure	Decreases contraction
Dilates coronary arteries	Constricts coronary arteries	
Lungs	Opens up airways	Closes airways
GI tract	Slows down peristalsis	Increases peristalsis
Sex	Allows male ejaculation	Allows male erection
Bladder	Contracts the bladder	Relaxes the bladder
Skin	Produces sweat	—
Constricts blood vessels		
Muscles	Constricts blood flow	—
Sweat	Increases	

they work together to permit actions such as normal sexual functioning and urination (see Table 7.1).

INTERACTIONS BETWEEN FIBROMYALGIA AND AN ABNORMALLY REGULATED ANS

How do the workings of the ANS relate to fibromyalgia? The SNS is underactive in fibromyalgia in the sense that an increased ratio of excitatory to inhibitory responses from central sensitization results in lower blood flow rates, leaky capillaries, at relatively low baseline blood pressure. In the spinal fluid, norepinephrine and neuropeptide Y (a neuropeptide similar to epinephrine that acts as a sensor for the ANS, increases appetite, and calms nerves) levels are decreased. *Tilt-table testing,* in which patients lie down and are tilted upward on an examining table, shows normal baseline pulse and blood pressure but an exaggerated rise in blood pressure in many fibromyalgia patients. Some fibromyalgia patients have *neurally mediated hypotension,* in which decreased sympathetic activity lowers blood pressure, leading to dizziness and fatigue. (See Chapter 13).

According to Dr. Daniel J. Clauw at the University of Michigan, the ANS control mechanisms are out of sync in certain patients with fibromyalgia. Sensors dilate the blood vessels in one area and constrict them in an adjacent region without reason or provocation. Termed *autonomic dysregulation,* or *dysautonomia,* this loss of autoregulatory or local control causes a variety of clinical problems associated with fibromyalgia.

How do the ANS sensors lose their fine-tuning control? As discussed in Chapter 4 and shown in Figure 7.1, autonomic signals are transmitted from the periphery by events such as physical trauma or changes in posture by myelinated

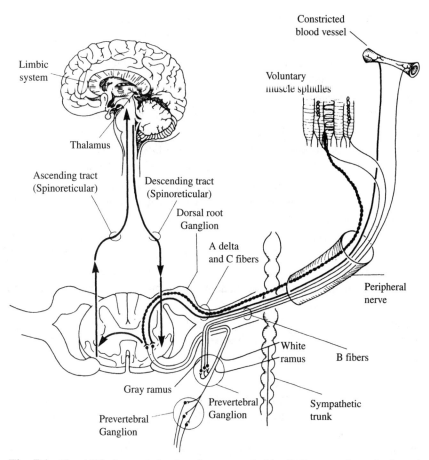

Fig. 7.1. *The ANS. Autonomic signals are carried by B fibers to the spinal cord and ascend to the limbic system of the brain via the spinoreticular tract.*

B fibers via a few detours to the spinal cord. From there the ANS ascends the spinal cord via the spinoreticular tract to the limbic system of the brain. In fibromyalgia, however, repeated incoming signals from unmyelinated C fibers to the dorsal horn of the spinal cord may also create nociceptor hypersensitivity. Further overwhelming sympathetic controls cause autonomic B fibers to carry messages usually carried by C fibers. Group B fibers are nerve fibers which are moderately myelinated (less than Group A and more than Group B). Nociceptive stimuli are now transmitted through normally nonnociceptive transmitters. This results in blood vessel constriction and hyperalgesia. When this leads to the appearance or sensation of swelling, it is called *neurogenic inflammation*. Here, sensory afferent end-organ stimuli cause SNS and neuropeptide release, which produces plasma extravasation, or swelling (edema). This swelling presses on small nerves and creates the sensation of numbness, burning, or tingling. Further, substance P can activate SNS receptors in the dorsal root ganglion. See Figure 13.2.

DYSAUTONOMIA ALLOWS FIBROMYALGIA TO MIMIC
AUTOIMMUNE DISEASES

Altered SNS tone can mimic immunologic or autoimmune disorders. Autoimmune disorders occur when the body becomes allergic to itself. Dysautonomia produces *reactive hyperemia,* or redness in the skin after palpation. This leads to a mottled appearance under the skin and can mimic or cause *dermatographia* (rubbing a key into the skin produces an impression that lasts for minutes), *livedo reticularis* (a red, lace-like, checkerboard appearance under the skin), and *Raynaud's phenomenon.* All of these features, particularly Raynaud's phenomenon (which is what happens when your fingers become patriotic by turning red, white, and blue when exposed to cold temperatures), are prominent features of autoimmune diseases such as systemic lupus erythematosus and scleroderma, which are also characterized by dysautonomia and neurogenic inflammation. One of the procedures used to diagnose systemic lupus is the lupus band test. In the early 1980s, some investigators reported that this skin biopsy was giving false-positive readings in fibromyalgia patients. Occasional deposits of small amounts of immune complexes (which give the false-positive result) were shown to result from leaky capillaries observed with autonomic dysfunction. We have seen patients erroneously diagnosed with lupus who really had fibromyalgia with dysautonomia.

THE CLINICAL SPECTRUM OF FIBROMYALGIA RESULTING
FROM DYSAUTONOMIA

Abnormal autonomic regulation leads to many secondary clinical syndromes that can be part of fibromyalgia or fall into the realm of *fibromyalgia-associated conditions.* Most of these conditions are discussed in detail in Chapters 13 and 14 and are listed in Table 7.2. They include mitral valve prolapse, noncardiac chest pain, migraine/tension headaches, irritable bowel syndrome (also called *spastic colitis* or *functional bowel syndrome*), premenstrual syndrome, and irritable bladder.

Infrequently, serious derangements of the ANS leads to prolonged stimulation of pain amplifiers, which results in chronic neurogenic inflammation. The most important complication of this is a condition of sympathetically mediated pain known as *reflex sympathetic dystrophy,* which is reviewed in Chapter 13.

It has been postulated that a hypervigilance is associated with dysautonomia, which results in fibromyalgia patients becoming acutely aware of normal bodily activities. Patients report being uncomfortable as they feel palpitations or experience spasm in the abdomen, or have difficulty tolerating daily noises.

Table 7.2. *Examples of Autonomic Dysfunction in Fibromyalgia*

Neurally mediated hypotension—abnormally low blood pressure
Mitral valve prolapse—causes palpitations due to release of epinephrine, which increases heart rates
Neurogenic inflammation—swelling on an autonomic basis
Reflex sympathetic dystrophy (Complex regional pain syndrome Type 1)—neurogenic inflammation with severe pain
Migraine headaches—autonomically mediated abnormal dilation of brain blood vessels
Numbness, tingling, burning—when abnormal vascular tone or neurogenic inflammation presses on nerves or activates their sensors
Livedo reticularis, Raynaud's and palmar erythema—loss of autonomic control in capillaries under the skin and increased flow through small, superficial arteries
Generalized hypervigilance—increased sympathetic activity
Neuro-otologic problems—dizziness, dry eyes and mouth
Loss of heart rate variability—due to stress of chronic autonomic activation

Heart Rate Variability

Seminal work by Dr. Martinez-Lavin in Mexico City and confirmed by others have allowed practitioners to assess autonomic nervous system function in fibromyalgia. It turns out that relentless hyperactivity of the sympathetic nervous system is worse at night, when the system fails to dimimish its excessive activity. As a consequence, there is less "heart rate variability," or increase in heart rate when a new stress is applied. This can be easily measured with a specialized heart monitor. Sympathetic hyperactivity is associated with increased presence and severity of chronic widespread pain.

SUMMING UP

Regulation of autonomic control may be abnormal in fibromyalgia. Autonomic dysregulation can mimic some features observed in autoimmune disease and is often mistaken for them. Many commonly observed complaints in fibromyalgia, such as irritable colon, mitral valve prolapse, edema, reddish discoloration of the skin, and tension headaches, are due in part to abnormalities of the ANS.

FOR FURTHER READING

Arnanson BGW. Autonomic regulation of immune function. In PA Low, ed. *Clinical Autonomic Disorders*. 2nd Ed. Philadelphia, PA: Lippincott-Raven; 1997: 147–159.

Bakarat A, Vogelzangs N, Licht CM, *et al*. Dysregulation of the autonomic nervous system and its association with the presence and intensity of chronic widespread pain. *Arthritis Care Res.* 2012; *64*: 1209–1216.

Littlejohn GO, Weinstein C, Helme RD. Increased neurogenic inflammation in fibrositis syndrome. *J Rheumatol 14*, 1987: 1022–1025.

Martinez-Lavin M, Hermosillo AG. Autonomic nervous system dysfunction may explain the multisystem features of fibromyalgia. *Seminars Arthritis Rheum* 2000; *29*: 197–199.

Martinez-Lavin M, Vargas A. Complex adaptive systems allostasis in fibromyalgia. *Rheum Dis Clin North Am.* 2009; *35*: 285–298.

Part III

HOW AND WHERE THE BODY CAN BE AFFECTED BY FIBROMYALGIA

I have been a frozen wretch my whole life, hardly able to stand a whiff of wind or pain...My rheumatic pains leave me no rest...I suffer stomach aches most of the time...My headaches are so terrible that life seems filled with bile...paralyzing fatigue...It is possible that I am more seriously ill than my doctors think. The pain will not go away.

Letters of Alfred Bernhard Nobel (1833–1896)

Fibromyalgia is known for its diversity of symptoms and signs. Every part of the body can be involved, and many of these manifestations are frequently misunderstood. This part discusses the more important symptoms and signs reported by fibromyalgia patients. Most of these complaints are complemented by case studies that illustrate the contexts in which they are most commonly encountered.

8
Generalized Complaints

Complaint is the largest tribute Heaven receives.

Jonathan Swift (1667–1745),
Thoughts on Various Subjects, 1711

Fibromyalgia is a syndrome rather than a disease, and as such has a variety of features. Any part of the body can be involved, especially when fibromyalgia is induced or aggravated by multiple factors. This chapter will review some of the generalized complaints expressed by fibromyalgia patients and place them in perspective.

CONSTITUTIONAL SYMPTOMS AND SIGNS

One of the major problems fibromyalgia sufferers encounter is difficulty communicating how they really feel. Complaints can be subjective and hard to verify or quantify. They consist of *symptoms,* or expressions of what is bothersome, and *signs*. Physical signs are observed during a physical examination, such as a rash or an irregular heartbeat, and are easier to validate. Constitutional symptoms or signs are generalized and do not belong to any specific organ system or region of the body, and are listed in Table 8.1.

FATIGUE

Jane was an anthropology graduate student. In addition to carrying a full load of classes, she moonlighted as a waitress 20 hours a week. This pace was maintained until Jane caught what seemed to be a bad case of flu with a sore throat, runny nose, cough, fever, aching, fatigue, and swollen glands. Although most of her flu symptoms disappeared after several weeks, Jane never felt the same. The fatigue and aching became more pronounced, and Jane had to quit her waitressing job. She forced herself to go to class and was so exhausted that she spent most weekends in bed. Despite all of the bed rest, Jane never slept well, and began noticing stiffness and spasm in her upper back and neck areas. The Student Health Service referred her to

Table 8.1. *Prevalence (%) of Frequently Observed Symptoms and Signs in Fibromyalgia Patients*

Widespread pain with tender points	100
Generalized weakness, muscle and joint aches	80
Unrefreshing sleep	75
Fatigue	75
Stiffness	70
Anxiety	60
Psychological stress	60
Dizziness/vertigo	55
Tension headache	55
Cognitive impairment, fibro "fog"	50
Painful periods	40
Irritable colon	40
Subjective numbness, burning, tingling	35
Subjective complaints of swelling or edema	35
Depression	35
Skin redness, lace-like skin mottling	30
Complaints of fever	20
Complaints of swollen glands	20
Complaints of non-medication dryness, dry eyes	18
Post-traumatic stress disorder	18
Nocturnal myoclonus, restless legs syndrome	15
Raynaud's	15
Irritable bladder, interstitial cystitis	12
Chronic pelvic pain	12
Reflex sympathetic dystrophy	5
Bipolar illness	5

an internist, who ordered tests, all of which were normal. Jane now paces herself with rest periods alternating with active ones, avoids daytime sleeping, takes cyclobenzaprine (Flexeril) two hours before retiring at night, and engages in a general conditioning program. Even though Jane is still unable to work, at least she did not have to drop out of school. Fatigue is still a major problem, but its level of intensity seems to be slowly diminishing.

As with Jane, generalized fatigue is a prominent feature of fibromyalgia. Between 60 and 80% of fibromyalgia patients complain of *fatigue,* which is defined as physical or mental exhaustion or weariness. However, there are many reasons for fatigue. In one survey, 20% of the women in the United States and 14% of the men rated themselves as being significantly fatigued. This feeling can come on like a wave or be continuous.

Some of the basic causes of fatigue include emotional stress, depression, physical illness, poor sleeping, and poor eating. Examples of fatigue-inducing conditions include working too hard, substance abuse, anemia, low thyroid level, side effects of medication, overtraining, menopause, pregnancy, diabetes, heart disease, kidney impairment, cancer, depression, excessive perfectionist tendencies, autoimmune disease, and inflammation.

The majority of patients with fibromyalgia and chronic, otherwise unexplained fatigue in whom a primary psychiatric diagnosis has been ruled out also meet the criteria for chronic fatigue syndrome (see Chapter 13).

DO FIBROMYALGIA PATIENTS RUN FEVERS?

Amber was having difficulty explaining what she meant. Until she was diagnosed as having fibromyalgia, she told doctors about her fevers. She related that it felt as if she was burning up or breaking out into a cold sweat. Physicians would obtain a normal temperature, look for infection, and inform her that they could not find anything. Although she never took her temperature during these episodes, Amber recalled her mother explaining that 97.4°F was normal for her and that when she had a temperature of 98.4°F it was a fever. Nobody believed her until a rheumatologist explained that altered sympathetic nervous system activity in fibromyalgia produces a feverish sensation. However, if her temperature was higher than 99.6°F on an ongoing basis, something other than fibromyalgia needed to be considered.

Everybody has a temperature, but few people run persistent fevers. A *fever* is defined as a body temperature above 99.6°F. Occasionally, patients complain to their doctor about recurrent fevers and relate that their baseline temperature is usually 96–97°F. Therefore, the normal temperature obtained at examination is a fever. Twenty percent of fibromyalgia patients include fevers in their list of complaints. Many, in fact, feel feverish. Hot and cold sweats or the sensation of "burning up" are not uncommon in fibromyalgia patients and reflect dysautonomia (see Chapter 7). Thirty percent with fibromyalgia relate some degree of cold intolerance. Verifiable, chronic fever is *not* a feature of primary fibromyalgia but an indication that another condition is causing fibromyalgia-like complaints. Inflammatory conditions, infections, and tumors should be sought out.

SWOLLEN OR TENDER GLANDS

The body's lymphatic system is a network of glands or lymph nodes that assist veins in clearing up water and debris and returning fluid from the arms, legs, and other areas of the body to the heart area. An infection such as a sore throat can lead to swollen lymph nodes in the neck area. Chronic poor circulation can produce edema from poor lymph drainage or varicose veins in the legs. Most lymph glands are enlarged when we have a local infection, an inflammation, or a malignancy.

Twenty percent of fibromyalgia patients complain of having swollen lymph nodes. Many who have a postinfectious fatigue syndrome start out with swollen glands, but the glands are no longer enlarged by the time a fibromyalgia specialist is consulted. Those who are thin also have relatively prominent lymph nodes, a condition not associated with any disease. As with a fever, if the doctor can feel the lymph nodes in a given area, this is not due to fibromyalgia but represents a circulation problem, allergic reaction, infection, inflammatory process, cancer, or simply bodily thinness.

The perception of tender lymph glands is common in fibromyalgia and reflects allodynia. The glands themselves are not enlarged or abnormal under the microscope.

FIBROMYALGIA CAN APPEAR DIFFERENT IN DIFFERENT AGE GROUPS AND GENDERS

When fibromyalgia appears in very young and elderly patients, it is not only uncommon but presents differently than expected. New-onset fibromyalgia in these age groups can be very difficult to diagnose.

Fibromyalgia in Childhood and Adolescence

Diana was every mother's dream. A 14-year-old girl from a comfortable middle-class family, she was an honor student, star of the volleyball team, and president of her church youth group. Diana never complained, was very serious, spent more time on her homework assignments than was necessary, and sometimes had difficulty relaxing. While serving at the volleyball championship, she felt a pop in her right shoulder, which swelled up a few hours later. The pain and swelling were not only uncomfortable but also very upsetting. Over the following weeks, Diana's shoulder seemed frozen and immovable and both of her hands became puffy, especially the right. Although the initial mechanical problem in her right shoulder slowly healed with physical therapy, Diana became very tired, achy, and depressed, had difficulty sleeping, and became aware of numerous tender points. A pediatric rheumatologist diagnosed her as having juvenile fibromyalgia with reflex sympathetic dystrophy. Diana was given ibuprofen and a few steroid injections into her shoulder, and a vigorous rehabilitation program was prescribed. Although the therapy was quite painful at first, Diana slowly responded to it. A psychologist working with the rehabilitation center taught her biofeedback, yoga, and relaxation techniques. Her perfectionistic tendencies were redirected in a more socially useful direction.

Whereas fibromyalgia is present in 2% of adults and is the third or fourth most common reason for seeking a rheumatology consultation, it is the twelfth most common reason for seeking a pediatric rheumatology evaluation. Pediatric rheumatologists see a new child or adolescent with fibromyalgia just a few times a year. There are probably fewer than 10,000 children in the United States with the syndrome, 90% of whom are adolescents. This has led some investigators to speculate that a hormonal connection may be very important. In addition to its relative rarity, preadult fibromyalgia is different from adult fibromyalgia. How so? In two ways: reflex sympathetic dystrophy (RSD) and a typical psychiatric profile.

Few centers have much experience with childhood fibromyalgia, but studies from Children's Hospital of Los Angeles suggest that a subset of adolescents with fibromyalgia fit a specific profile. An example could be a 10- to 15-year old girl who has grown up as a "perfect, model" child, never complains, and has perfectionistic tendencies and excellent grades (but is often home schooled) in school. They appear mature beyond their years, and meet the needs of others at their own expense. Mom frequently acts as the spokesperson at the rheumatology consultation.

A seemingly trivial sports injury or emotional event (e.g., a move, divorce, change in nuclear family, change in school or friends) can be followed by widespread pain and fatigue. Splinting or casting the injured area is of no benefit and "growing pains" simply don't get better. Additionally, reflex sympathetic dystrophy with swelling of both upper extremities (more severe on one side than on the other), inability to move an arm or shoulder, and mottling changes in the skin is often present. RSD is found in 1–10% of adult fibromyalgia patients but is seen in 20–40% of adolescents. Adolescents with severe growing pains, disturbed sleep, irritable colon, attention deficit, and hypermobile (very limber) joints frequently develop full-blown fibromyalgia in adulthood.

Unlike adult fibromyalgia, the juvenile syndrome responds only minimally to tricyclic antidepressants and pain medication. The best results correlate with intensive, vigorous physical therapy and exercise, steroid injections to affected areas or intermittent courses of oral steroids, and psychological support. Even though the presentation of fibromyalgia in young people is more severe than in adults, children and adolescents have a better prognosis than many adults. If the treatment program outlined above is aggressively pursued, 80% of young patients have substantial resolution of the syndrome within two to three years.

Fibromyalgia in the Elderly

Wilma starting fading after her 70th birthday. She began complaining of aching in her middle and upper back areas, in addition to stiffness in her wrists and hands. Wilma's doctor performed blood tests that showed a slightly elevated sedimentation rate, which could signify inflammation. Dr. Lear was not sure whether this was polymyalgia rheumatica, a common joint disease among senior citizens, or early rheumatoid arthritis. Wilma also had fatigue, tension headaches, and difficulty sleeping. However, Dr. Lear seemed so busy and rushed that she was too intimidated to take up his valuable time by reporting these symptoms, which she thought were less important. Wilma was given low-dose prednisone, 10 mg a day, which helped greatly during the first week. Over the following month, her symptoms worsened and Wilma became anxious and panicky. Dr. Lear referred her to Dr. Green, who took a more detailed history. In the last year Wilma had lost her son, been involved in an automobile accident, and caught a bad flu; her best friend had had a serious stroke. Dr. Green diagnosed her as having fibromyalgia, tapered her steroids, referred her to a gerontology patient support center, and prescribed low-dose bedtime nortriptyline (Pamelor), an antidepressant that promotes restful sleep.

As patients with long-standing fibromyalgia age, the syndrome usually persists. Many female patients report that menopause modestly decreases their symptoms. But can people over the age of 65 develop fibromyalgia-like symptoms? Since this is an unusual event, the differential diagnosis reviewed earlier in this chapter should be considered. This applies especially to hypothyroidism, Sjogren's syndrome (dry eyes, dry mouth, aching, and fatigue), rheumatoid arthritis, occult malignancy, and polymyalgia rheumatica. A normal sedimentation rate, negative ANA (antinuclear antibody), negative rheumatoid factor, and normal TSH (thyroid test) usually allow doctors to make a definitive diagnosis of fibromyalgia. Studies of patients with older-onset fibromyalgia show fewer functional symptoms such as anxiety, stress, or unrefreshed sleep, and more musculoskeletal complaints than their younger counterparts. Polymyalgia rheumatica is far more common than late-onset fibromyalgia. It presents with aching in the upper back, neck, buttocks, or thighs, along with a markedly elevated sedimentation rate. Many healthy older people have modestly elevated sedimentation rates. As a consequence, up to 40% of late-onset fibromyalgia patients in one survey were given corticosteroids before a correct diagnosis was made. Older-onset fibromyalgia is managed the same way as in younger adults. Finally, joint and muscle aches can be symptomatic of primary depression; this possibility always warrants careful consideration.

Fibromyalgia in Men

Since 90% of patients with fibromyalgia are females, does the syndrome differ in males? Men with fibromyalgia tend to have more severe symptoms, poorer physical functioning, and a lower quality of life. Hormones probably play a role in pain perception. It has been suggested that healthy males make 40% less serotonin than healthy women. We are not quite sure what this means, but even though women have lower tender point pain thresholds, men complain of "hurting all over" more often.

FOR FURTHER READING

Siegel DM, Janeway D, Baum J. Fibromyalgia syndrome in children and adolescents: Clinical features at presentation and status at follow up. *Pediatrics 101*, 1998: 377–382.

Yunus M, Masi AT, Calabro JJ, *et al.* Primary fibromyalgia (fibrositis): Clinical study of 50 patients with matched normal controls. *Semin Arthritis Rheum* 1981; *11*: 151–171.

Yunus MB, Inanici F, Aldag JC, Mangold RF. Fibromyalgia in men: Comparison of clinical features with women. *J Rheumatol* 2000; *31*: 2464–2467.

Wallace DJ The fibromyalgia syndrome. *Ann Med 29*, 1997: 9–21.

9

"I'm Stiff and Achy"—Musculoskeletal Complaints

I don't deserve this award, but I have arthritis and I don't deserve that either.

Jack Benny (1894–1974)

Patients with each of the 150 distinct rheumatic disorders frequently have overlapping muscle and joint complaints. Weakness, myalgias, arthralgias, spasm, lack of endurance, and stiffness are prominent features of fibromyalgia that may be difficult to differentiate from other conditions. The prominence of complaints in this area is what frequently brings patients to a musculoskeletal specialist such as a rheumatologist, as opposed to an infectious disease expert, general internist, or endocrinologist.

MUSCLE FINDINGS: WEAKNESS, MYALGIAS, LACK OF ENDURANCE, AND SPASM

Abigail was devastated after the unexpected death of her younger brother at age 30. Her physical and mental health had seemed tenuous, but she managed to pull herself together for the funeral and the visits of relatives from the Midwest. When it was over, Abigail's coping skills began to fray. First, she began experiencing left-sided upper back pain and thought it was from lifting Aunt Minnie's suitcase when taking her to the airport. Abigail saw the chiropractor she had consulted three or four times over a five-year period for similar backaches. However, this time the pain did not go away and spread to the right side. Dr. Johnson's manipulations usually "snapped things back into place," but this time they made her worse. Abigail became very concerned when her fiancee tried to take her to Myrtle Beach for a relaxing weekend and found that she was in agony whenever he hugged her. Although she had been an aerobics instructor, Abigail found it very difficult to do her morning exercise routine and after several weeks gave up. Trying to exercise was extremely painful. Innocent movements such as washing her back in the shower caused her muscles to tighten up and go into spasm.

Dr. Johnson referred her to a rheumatologist, who diagnosed fibromyalgia and instituted a medication, education, and rehabilitation program.

Over 80% of fibromyalgia patients have muscular symptoms or signs. Aching in the muscles, or *myalgias,* is common in the upper or lower back and neck area. Myalgias are usually present on both the right and left sides and present as a dull, throbbing discomfort. *Spasm,* defined as an involuntary muscular contraction, is less common than the sense of tightness in muscles that seems like spasm. Muscular aches tend to worsen after exercise and activity and as the day wears on. The discomfort is generally more severe in the late afternoons and feels "flu-like."

What is going on in the muscles? As discussed in Chapter 5, the muscles are weak only if deconditioning is present. Areas of taut bands may be felt as tender points. Some fibromyalgia patients who once engaged in vigorous exercise complain that they feel exhausted after a short workout and no longer have endurance. How does this happen? Postexertional pain occurs when arteries in the muscle constrict and not enough oxygen gets to these areas. Exercise requires increased oxygen to the muscles, and the lack of oxygen produces muscle pain. Fibromyalgia patients don't use oxygen optimally and prematurely deplete their energy reserves. This leads to deconditioning and produces a vicious cycle that promotes a fear of exercise.

Myalgias should be differentiated from inflammation of the muscles, which is known as *myositis,* and other conditions associated with aching muscles. Inflammatory processes such as polymyositis or systemic lupus can mimic fibromyalgia, as can a low thyroid blood level, myasthenia gravis, multiple sclerosis, infections, and anemia. Common prescription medications infrequently induce side effects affecting muscles, which leads to aching or weakness. Examples of this include certain cholesterol-lowering preparations (e.g., lovastatin [Mevacor], atorvastatin [Lipitor], pravastatin [Pravachol]) and the gout medicine colchicine. Inflammatory myositis, hypothyroidism, and the above-mentioned drugs can produce abnormally high blood levels of the muscle enzyme *creatine phosphokinase* (CPK) or abnormal electrical tracings in muscles on an electromyogram (EMG). Sometimes patients with primary muscle disorders have fibromyalgia-like complaints that can be diagnosed only with a muscle biopsy.

SOFT TISSUE AND JOINT COMPLAINTS: WIDESPREAD PAIN, ARTHRALGIAS, AND STIFFNESS

Janice was sure she had arthritis. Her mother could always tell when it was going to rain, and now Janice seemed to have this meteorologic prowess. As the day progressed, she would feel as if her body was stiffening up. Janice began noticing aching with pain in her shoulders and the back of her neck, particularly if she was premenstrual or had slept poorly. Janice felt much older than her 40 years. Her family doctor could not find any evidence of arthritis on examination or blood testing, and X-rays of her neck and shoulders were normal. Ibuprofen was prescribed, bringing temporary relief. Ultimately, it was concluded that Janice had a mild form of fibromyalgia that became evident when the weather changed, just before her period, and when she did not get enough sleep. Janice takes cyclobenzaprine (Flexeril) about three or four times a month when the discomfort starts to interfere with her ability to do things, but generally she feels well.

The International Association for the Study of Pain has defined *pain* as an unpleasant sensory and emotional experience. Widespread pain (from pain amplification) is such a prominent feature of fibromyalgia syndrome that it is included in the definition of the syndrome. The pain usually emanates from the soft tissues, muscles, and joints. Soft tissues include the supporting structures of joints such as tendons, bursae, and ligaments, as well as the myofascia. The myofascia lies between the lower skin (dermis) and muscles and consists of connective tissue and fat, which buffer muscles and provide structural integrity and support. The nature of the pain is highly variable. Some patients use descriptive terms such as *aching, burning, gnawing, smarting,* or *throbbing.* Pain can change sites and often gets better or worse on its own. Tender points are common in myofascial planes.

Fibromyalgia does not damage or inflame joints, but it can produce joint complaints. More than 80% of patients with fibromyalgia describe symptoms of aching in their joints, or *arthralgias,* and 60% have stiffness. Many patients also have other forms of arthritis, especially osteoarthritis, and a few have autoimmune disorders such as lupus or rheumatoid arthritis with a secondary fibromyalgia.

A form of neck osteoarthritis, or being born with a narrow spinal canal, can lead to cervical spinal stenosis. This tightening of the spinal canal in the neck can be detected on an MRI scan and may aggravate the symptoms of fibromyalgia. Unlike degenerative osteoarthritis or rheumatoid arthritis, the arthralgias are not located primarily in the small joints of the hands or feet. In fibromyalgia, symptoms are usually prominent in the upper back, neck, shoulder, and hip areas. Sometimes, patients who present with low back pain really have fibromyalgia. Tender points in the buttock can be mistaken for disc disease. Other parts of the body, especially those that have been overused, can be involved.

Whereas morning stiffness is an important feature of osteoarthritis and rheumatoid arthritis, most fibromyalgia patients become stiff in the late afternoon and early evening or when they have been in one position for a prolonged period of time. Stiffness is a difficult sensation to convey to others. Rheumatologists use the term *gelling* to denote the "jello"-like feeling of the stiff, tightened joints, muscles, and soft tissues of fibromyalgia. It improves when you move around, apply heat, or take a hot shower.

Soft Tissue Discomfort with a Mass: The Fibromyalgia Nodule

A large number of fibromyalgia patients have "nodules" or areas under the skin that feel like a small ball or "taut band." Soft tissues include the supporting structures of joints such as tendons, bursae, and ligaments, as well as the myofascia. The ACR tender points represent the most frequent areas of myofascial discomfort. The presence of "nodules" is common in some of the upper back and lower neck regions. They tend to be firm, mobile, globular or spindle-shaped tender structures consisting of fatty tissue, fibrous cords and muscles. Inflammation is not present.

Hypermobility

Some reports suggest an association between benign hypermobility syndrome and FM. Patients with this condition can do amazing things, such as touching their thumb to their forearm, twisting their ankle around itself, and extending their elbows and knees beyond 180 degrees. Hypermobile patients tend to dislocate tendons and ligaments more easily and develop earlier onset osteoarthritis.

FOR FURTHER READING

McBeth J, Jones K. Epidemiology of chronic musculoskeletal pain. *Best Pract Res Clin Rheumatol.* 2007 Jun; *21*(3): 403–425.

Sendur OF, Odabasi BB, Turan Y. The overlooked diagnosis in rheumatology: Benign joint hypermobility syndrome. *J Musculoskeletal Pain* 2010; *18*: 277–287.

10

Tingles, Shocks, Wires, and Neurologic Complaints

The brain is a wonderful organ. It starts working the moment you get up in the morning, and does not stop until you get into the office.

Robert Frost (1874–1963)

Even though headaches, sleep disorders, cognitive impairment, burning, numbness, and tingling are potentially debilitating features of fibromyalgia, very few patients first consult a neurologist when they develop what turn out to be fibromyalgia symptoms. It has become apparent that the central, peripheral, and autonomic nervous systems play a more important role in fibromyalgia than was previously thought. This section will focus on these complaints and what causes them.

HEADACHE

Colleen had a splitting headache. Her temples were throbbing, and she could barely concentrate. When Dr. Smith prescribed Fioricet (acetaminophen with caffeine and butalbital), not only did the headache disappear but some discomfort in her upper and lower back that she had never bothered to complain about did also. Over the next few months, Colleen needed Fioricet almost daily. Whenever she stopped taking it, the headaches returned with a vengeance. Dr. Smith referred her to a neurologist, who diagnosed Colleen as having fibromyalgia with associated "muscular contraction tension headaches." Colleen was told that the caffeine and barbiturate in Fioricet helped her headaches in the short term but that continuous use resulted in "rebound" headaches from aspirin, caffeine, and barbiturate withdrawal. The neurologist stopped all her medication and helped Colleen ride out the withdrawal. She prescribed amitriptyline (Elavil) at bedtime for headache protection, and Colleen is now much improved.

Most fibromyalgia patients complain of recurrent headaches. These headaches usually are one of two types: tension or migraine.

Muscular Contraction, or Tension Headaches

Tension headaches are muscular contraction headaches. Patients describe these headaches as a dull "tight band around the head" similar to what they feel in other muscles of the body. A sustained muscle contraction can compress small vessels in the area. Tension headaches and migraines are often associated with low elevations of substance P levels and decreased serotonin levels, stress, and low cellular pH (a more acidic cellular environment).

Tension headaches frequently involve the forehead, jaw, and temple areas. Occipital headaches, or pain in the upper part of the back of the neck, can be a type of tension headache and are associated with muscle spasm or stiffness. Osteoarthritis of the cervical spine can also cause occipital headaches. On occasion, moving the neck in any direction is painful. Tension headaches usually respond to the same remedies used to treat myalgias, arthralgias, and spasm.

Migraine Headaches

Ten percent of the U.S. population suffers from vascular-mediated migraine headaches. Usually one-sided, associated with light sensitivity (photophobia), manifested by pounding, and preceded by a premonition of coming on, migraines occur in 20% of patients with fibromyalgia. Low serotonin levels are found in migraine sufferers, which in turn can alter vascular tone. Physiologically, a migraine begins with constriction of blood vessels (which produces the premonition, or aura) followed by dilation. When arteries dilate, the stretching of the blood vessels and nerves evokes an intense headache.

Migraines are much more common in fibromyalgia patients who have ANS dysfunction. They complain of a throbbing or aching on one side of the head. This can be coupled with nausea or vomiting, visual disturbance (ocular migraine), or dizziness. Migraines can be brought on by unpleasant emotional stress, certain foods, menstruation, weather changes, smoke, hunger, or fatigue.

SLEEP ABNORMALITIES: NONRESTORATIVE SLEEP, SLEEP MYOCLONUS, BRUXISM

The alarm clock rang at 6 A.M., and Deidre felt as though she had never slept, even though she went to bed at 10 P.M. the evening before. She forced herself up and got ready for work. Deidre felt exhausted. This was happening with increasing frequency. Her initial response was anger—which she kept to herself. This seemed to tighten her head and neck muscles even more. That evening, Deidre decided to have two screwdrivers (vodka with orange juice) with dinner. She passed out at 9 P.M. and fell into a deep sleep. However, at 2 A.M. she awakened with palpitations and felt wired. Unable to get back to sleep, she made an appointment with her physician. Dr. Jones explained that nonrefreshing sleep is a common feature of fibromyalgia and that alcohol usually makes the problem worse, as does keeping anger to oneself. Deidre was given a prescription for nortriptyline (Pamelor) and joined the Arthritis Foundation, where she enrolled in their Fibromyalgia Self-Help course.

Sleep is necessary to promote the production of chemicals important in tissue growth and maintenance of immune function. As was mentioned in Chapter 6, nonrestorative (or nonrefreshing) sleep is found in most fibromyalgia patients. We all go through four stages of sleep, ranging from light to deep, where brain waves are denoted by the Greek letters alpha, beta, gamma, and delta. Persistent alpha wave intrusion into slow delta wave sleep results in waking up feeling sore all over and sometimes feeling more tired than when going to bed. Fibromyalgia patients make less growth hormone (which has little to do with growing in adults but is essential to maintain certain body functions) than healthy people while asleep, which can accelerate muscle injury and increase pain levels. These electrical abnormalities can be documented with a brain wave sleep study, known as a polysomnogram or a sleep electroencephalogram, which has been demonstrated in Figure 6.2. Patients with sleep disorders and fibromyalgia also might have cardiopulmonary disease, be smokers, have a cough, or drink increased amounts of caffeine or alcohol which need to be considered in the equation.

Restless Legs Syndrome

Restless legs syndrome may be present in up to 10% of the United States population, but has been reported in 15–50% with FM. A form of *periodic limb movement syndrome* and also known as *sleep myoclonus*, patients complain of a sudden jerking, lifting, shooting out or movement in their legs during sleep and relief with movement. Men and women are equally affected, with onset between the ages of 40 and 60 most of the time. Individuals are often alerted to this sleep behavior by their bed partners. Patients can feel a need to move their legs, which is relieved by moving or walking. Manifested electrically as an alpha-wave burst followed by limb movement, restless leg syndrome sufferers have excess sympathetic tone, dopamine deficiency, possible iron deficiency, and hypoxia, as well as more movement arousals and less stage 3 and 4 sleep. They are less responsive to usually prescribed sleep medications, but often do well with massage, cold compresses, iron, dopaminergic remedies (e.g., pramipexole [Mirapex]), quinine, or clonazepam (Klonopin).

Bruxism

Temporomandibular joint dysfunction syndrome is a regional manifestation of myofascial discomfort that is also a feature of FM. Most of these patients grind their teeth and bruxism is a manifestation of this syndrome associated with compromised sleep.

COGNITIVE IMPAIRMENT OR "BRAIN FATIGUE"

Esther is a professional fundraiser whose mild fibromyalgia had been generally under good control. Friends and co-workers marveled at her ability to remember dates, phone numbers, and the names of everybody's spouses and children. Over the last few months, however, Esther had occasional difficulty recalling quickly some of the obscure facts that were her trademark. What amazed her was that nobody could tell the difference. Since her mother suffered from Alzheimer's disease, Esther consulted her mother's neurologist to make sure she did not have an early case. Her neurologic exam and an MRI scan of her brain were normal. Dr. Chapman ordered a single photon emission computed tomography (SPECT) scan, which suggested that some parts of the brain were not getting as much oxygen as they should. This reflected an abnormality in ANS regulation of blood vessel tone. Esther was told to pace herself during the day, with periods of activity alternating with four 20-minute rest periods, and was reassured. Dr. Chapman told her that if she did not improve, he could give her a low dose of fluoxetine (Prozac) and prescribe a cognitive therapy rehabilitation program.

Some of our fibromyalgia patients are concerned because they cannot think clearly, remember names and dates, balance their checkbook, or add numbers the way they once did. Characterized by confusion, memory blanks, word mix-ups, and concentration difficulties, these changes are often subtle and imperceptible to the physician who hears the complaint. Cognitive impairment, which some patients term "brain fatigue" or "fibrofog," is found in 20% of fibromyalgia patients. These complaints may be fleeting, intermittent, or constant, and until recently were attributed to depression or stress. Additionally, some patients describe dizziness (which is not movement related), clumsiness and dropping things (which are not part of neurologic diseases such as multiple sclerosis), or visual changes or eye pain (which are not part of migraines). If these concerns are not handled wisely, patients are more likely to secondarily develop anxiety, panic, mood swings, and irritability (but not more pain).

Is Cognitive Dysfunction Real, and How Can We Test for It?

For years, rheumatologists were as guilty as other doctors of ascribing cognitive impairment to depression or stress. How else could they explain the normal findings on neurologic examinations, MRI scans of the brain, and spinal fluid tests? However, on the basis of recently published work, we now know that cognitive impairment is real, and we are working hard to educate our colleagues.

Two lines of evidence provide support for the concept of nonpsychological cognitive dysfunction that are reviewed in Chapter 4. First, in Chapter 6 we discussed the role of cytokines, chemicals that induce cognitive impairment along with fibromyalgia. ANS abnormalities occasionally may produce enough spasm in cerebral blood vessels to deprive regions of the brain of oxygen. Interestingly, nonrestorative sleep by itself can produce functional brain imaging abnormalities.

Serious, obvious cognitive dysfunction is uncommon, found in less than 5% of fibromyalgia Patients.

NUMBNESS, BURNING, AND TINGLING

Frank managed a tire store that recently became computerized. He spent two-three hours a day "on-line" checking inventory and cash flow. When Frank began complaining of numbness and tingling in his hands, a co-worker suggested that it could be carpal tunnel syndrome. He consulted an orthopedist, who gave him a wrist splint and injected the carpal tunnel region with steroids. This was temporarily helpful. When Frank had his annual physical with Dr. Grant, he told her about the numbness and tingling in his hands but also mentioned that his feet felt numb at times as well. Dr. Grant's examination revealed normal pulses and neurologic findings, but some tenderness was elicited to palpation of the upper back, buttocks, and neck area. Dr. Grant ordered an EMG and a nerve conduction test, which were normal. Since diabetes, a herniated disc, vascular disease, and carpal tunnel syndrome were ruled out, Dr. Grant diagnosed Frank as having myofascial pain syndrome with neuralgia. After two weeks of taking low-dose amitriptyline (Elavil) and changing the position of his computer keyboard, the numbness was gone.

At some time, one-third of fibromyalgia patients will become aware of a vague sensation of numbness, tingling, or burning. These symptoms may be reported in any part of the body and tend to come and go. When neurologists are consulted, their physical findings are usually within normal limits. Muscle and nerve blood tests are also normal. Although diagnostic electrical evaluations with an EMG or a nerve conduction study can identify cervical or lumbar disc problems, diabetes or other metabolic abnormalities, inflammation, or compressive lesions such as carpal tunnel syndrome, these studies are normal in primary fibromyalgia.

Carpal tunnel syndrome consists of compression of the median nerve at the wrist as it enters the palm of the hand. Its prevalence is increased among fibromyalgia patients, especially those who work with computers all day and others with poor workstation body mechanics. Carpal tunnel syndrome is usually treated by splinting, local steroid injections, and, if needed, an occupational or physical therapy evaluation. Anybody suspected of having carpal tunnel syndrome should have a confirmatory median sensory nerve conduction study of the upper extremity before undergoing corrective surgery. Since hand numbness is a feature of *both* fibromyalgia and carpal tunnel syndrome, some patients have had expensive and unnecessary surgery that fails to relieve the numbness and tingling of fibromyalgia. Unfortunately, we have observed the distinctive scar on the inside surface of the wrist indicating carpal tunnel surgery in about 10% of our patients, many of whom did not require surgery.

What Causes Painful Nerve Sensations in Fibromyalgia?

Why should numbness and tingling be a feature of fibromyalgia? Painful nerve sensations are a mild form of neurogenic inflammation or local nerve compression caused by autonomic dysfunction. Unless reflex sympathetic dystrophy is present (see Chapter 13), it should evoke little concern. Although annoying and a cause of aggravated poor sleep, fibromyalgia neuralgia (painful nerve symptoms) never causes paralysis, strokes, or deformity. The management of numbness, tingling and burning is reviewed in Part VII, but the standard first-line therapy consists of tricyclic antidepressants such as amitriptyline (Elavil), or the anticonvulsant, gabapentin (Neurontin).

DRY EYES AND OTHER EYE OR EAR COMPLAINTS

Dry eyes or dry mouth, also known as *sicca symptoms,* have been reported in 10–35% of fibromyalgia patients. Manifested by burning, stinging, and redness of the eyes, and verified by pits in the cornea on a Rose Bengal or Lissamine green stain, diminished tearing in fibromyalgia has been attributed to altered autonomic nervous system activity. These small, difficult-to-see pits occur when the cornea does not receive enough moisture. Dry eyes are much more common than dry mouth.

Sicca related to fibromyalgia should be differentiated from an autoimmune mediated dry eyes, dry mouth, and arthritis condition known as *Sjogren's syndrome,* in which autoantibodies are usually present. In Sjogren's syndrome, viral infections (as in HIV or the mumps), alcoholism, and metabolic illnesses, the parotid (salivary) gland within the cheeks may become enlarged. Since tricyclic antidepressants are one of the principal treatments for fibromyalgia, and frequently cause dry eyes and dry mouth, it is sometimes difficult to ascertain how many people truly have fibromyalgia syndrome-induced dryness syndrome.

WHY AM I DIZZY? WHY DO NORMAL NOISES BOTHER ME?

More patients with fibromyalgia complain of feeling dizzy than otherwise healthy people. Dizziness can be a result of a bone spur in the neck causing pressure on the blood supply of the brain, chronic allergies with sinus inflammation, migraine, low blood pressure, medications, palpitations from autonomically mediated mitral valve prolapse, or a thyroid imbalance. Some fibromyalgia patients without these problems also notice a sensation of dizziness. Studies have suggested that the vestibular, or equilibrium, center in the ears is not optimally regulated in fibromyalgia patients. The reason is not well understood, but it may have to do with autonomic lack of blood flow to the vestibular center. Some fibromyalgia patients may have a low frequency nerve-mediated hearing loss that is asymptomatic. Recent evidence suggests that these fibromyalgia patients are not really dizzy. Dizziness is a sensation of being in motion, but what some fibromyalgia patients are experiencing is *vertigo,* a malfunction of the vestibular center of the ear producing a sensation that everything around you is in motion. There are more balance problems and falls. Some fibromyalgia patients have decreased noise tolerance on the basis of a hypervigilant vestibular reaction. Chemicals can also elicit stimuli that sensitize the limbic system (See Chapters 4 and 7) through "limbic kindling," which facilitates behavioral, autonomic, hormonal, and immune functions, producing "dizziness." Additionally, some fibromyalgia therapies, such as nonsteroidal anti-inflammatory drugs (NSAIDs), can lead to complaints of ringing in the ears, or *tinnitus,* or rarely, in other patients, diminished hearing. Increased sensitivity to bright lights or loud noises likely represents a global sensory hyperactivity. Some patients have had "syncopal" (passing out) reactions and dizziness, again perhaps in part due to the known overlap with neurally mediated hypotension (persistent low blood pressure associated with fatigue), or postural orthostatic tachycardia syndrome, or *POTS,* which is a form of dysautonomia.

FOR FURTHER READING

Gaisser ME, Glass JM, Rajcevska LD, *et al.* A psychological study of auditory and pressure sensitivity in patients with fibromyalgia and healthy controls, *J Pain* 2008; *9*: 417–422.

Kwiatek R, Barnden L, Tedman R, Jarrett R, *et al.* Regional cerebral blood flow in fibromyalgia. *Arthritis Rheum 43*, 2000: 2823–2833.

Mountz JM, Bradley LA, Modell J. G., *et al.* Fibromyalgia in women: Abnormalities of regional cerebral blood flow in the thalamus and the caudate nucleus are associated with low pain threshold levels. *Arthritis Rheum 38*, 1995: 926–938.

Williams DA, Clauw DJ, Glass JM, Perceived cognitive dysfunction in fibromyalgia syndrome, *J Musculoskeletal Pain* 2011; *19*: 66–75.

11

Insights into Insides: Chest, Cardiovascular, and Other Concerns

The human heart is like a ship on a stormy sea driven about by winds blowing from all four corners of heaven.

Martin Luther (1483–1546),
Preface to Psalms, 1534

Although some patients are concerned that their critical organs are involved in fibromyalgia, chest area symptoms infrequently are related to heart or lung disease. Palpitations, noncardiac chest pain, and subjective swelling or edema are important symptoms and signs of fibromyalgia. Reflux from the esophagus, gastrointestinal complaints, and female organ-related problems are also reviewed in this chapter in the context of fibromyalgia-associated concerns.

PALPITATIONS

The pounding in her chest was becoming unbearable, and Georgia was sure she would pass out. The sensation had been noticed before, but it usually stopped after several seconds. After several minutes, Georgia no longer felt lightheaded or dizzy. She broke into a cold sweat and heaved a sigh of relief. Her internist was aware of Georgia's intermittent musculoskeletal aches and spasms and fatigue, which were managed with ibuprofen and occasional gabapentin (Neurontin) at night. When Georgia mentioned her fatigue to Dr. Baker, her comments were greeted with silence and not immediately pursued. Consequently, she drank four Diet Cokes to make it through the workday in addition to her morning coffee. Dr. Baker ordered a two-dimensional echocardiogram (a heart image in ultrasound) that demonstrated evidence of mitral valve prolapse. He told Georgia that the palpitations were brought on by drinking too much caffeine, and said that if she could not reduce her caffeine intake substantially, he would have to prescribe a beta-blocker to control her heart rate.

The sense of having extra heartbeats, or *palpitations,* is reported in 10–20% of patients with fibromyalgia. Although heart disease, caffeine intake, anxiety, and other factors are associated with palpitations, many otherwise healthy young women have *mitral valve prolapse.* The prevalence of mitral valve prolapse is clearly increased in fibromyalgia. The mitral valve, one of the four valves of the heart that lies between its right-sided chambers, can become more floppy under ANS influence and produce palpitations. Patients feel as though they will pass out but rarely do. Mitral valve prolapse is also associated with chest pains and shortness of breath and can be easily diagnosed by a heart ultrasound known as a *two-dimensional echocardiogram.* Most patients with mitral valve prolapse do not require medication, and benefit from avoiding caffeine and learning how to relax. However, between 5–10% of these patients are referred to a cardiologist because they have potentially serious heart irregularities and may benefit from the initiation of heart drugs known as *beta-blockers.*

COSTOCHONDRITIS AND NONCARDIAC CHEST PAIN

Hannah's father died from a heart attack when he was 50 and her favorite aunt at 46. Her serum cholesterol was a bit high, and she was 20 pounds overweight. Soon after Hannah celebrated her 45th birthday and was promoted to a high-pressure but prestigious position as head of sales for a cosmetics firm, it happened. Hannah developed chest pains and neck spasms so severe that she was sure the end was near. Her family rushed her to a community hospital. Hannah's electrocardiogram, chest X-ray, blood count, and chemistry panel were normal. However, her pain did not go away with nitroglycerine or Zantac. When the doctor touched Hannah's third left rib at its juncture with the sternum (breast bone), she saw stars. Diagnosed as having costochondritis along with stress-induced fibromyalgia, Hannah was referred to an internist/rheumatologist for ongoing care.

As in Hannah's case, there is no question that costochondritis can be scary. The sternum, or breastbone, is connected to ribs by a ropelike tethering tissue. When this tissue (known as the *costochondral margin)* becomes irritated, it causes discomfort, especially in smokers, persons with lung disease or large breasts, and persons with inflammatory disorders such as rheumatoid arthritis. As noted in Figures 2.1 and 11.1, the costochondral margins are two of the tender points found in fibromyalgia. Sometimes referred to as *Tietze's syndrome,* this irritation produces chest pains. It sometimes takes an emergency room visit by a patient who is concerned about possibly having a heart attack before fibromyalgia is ultimately diagnosed. Costochondritis can be differentiated from cardiac pain because even though the sternum-rib attachments are tender to the touch, palpating the center of the sternum does not produce pain. A doctor may order chest or rib X-rays to make sure that there is no fracture.

Sometimes, patients with fibromyalgia report that it hurts when they take a deep breath. They fear it might be *pleurisy,* or irritation of the lining of the lung,

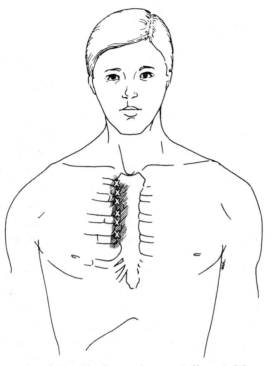

Fig. 11.1. *Costochondritis. The Xs mark potentially painful areas where ribs attach to the sternum.*

which is extremely common in autoimmune diseases. Hannah did not have pleurisy, but this complaint reflects abnormalities in respiratory muscles that connect the ribs or irritation of the intercostal nerves located in that area.

Another form of noncardiac chest pain relates to the *esophagus* and is discussed in Chapter 13.

DOCTOR, CAN'T YOU SEE HOW SWOLLEN I AM?

Iris had been diagnosed with fibromyalgia. Premenstrually, her muscle and joint aches worsened and she gained three to five pounds. Over a three-year period, Iris complained to several doctors that she felt swollen all the time. However, none of them found evidence of edema using the methods taught in medical school. One doctor bluntly and coldly told her that she was not swollen. A sympathetic internist prescribed Dyazide, a mild diuretic. Iris's fluid retention immediately lessened, but whenever she failed to take the medication, after several days her edema rebounded and became worse than ever. While on Dyazide, her muscle aching and spasms worsened. Her rheumatologist prescribed duloxetine (Cymbalta) for Iris's musculo-skeletal aches, which resulted in an additional ten-pound weight gain. Ultimately, Iris was weaned off both medications.

One area of conflict we have observed between doctors and fibromyalgia patients involves the physician's skepticism that a fluid retention problem is really present. Women with fibromyalgia frequently report fluid retention and swelling. However, physical examinations and routine testing usually fail to document objective swelling. When doctors respond instinctively and prescribe a diuretic, or water pill, the fibromyalgia worsens because these preparations mobilize fluid by promoting muscle actions that induce more pain. Too many of these patients unfortunately become dependent on diuretics and gain five–ten pounds within days when a different doctor or the patient stops the drug. Tricyclics in higher doses, particularly doxepin (Sinequan), duloxetine (Cymbalta), as well as the anticonvulsants gabapentin (Neurontin) and pregabalin (Lyrica) can cause fluid retention as well.

Research from Great Britain has suggested that there is subclinical swelling, or fluid retention that is not noticeable on classic palpation, an electrocardiogram, chest X-ray, or pitting on physical examination. These studies provide evidence that in fibromyalgia autonomically mediated sympathetic nervous system hypofunction induces neurogenic vasodilatation (see Chapter 7). This leads to decreased arterial vessel tone, which produces decreased capillary flow and results in increased capillary leakage of sodium and water. The net result is a perceived loss of volume by the kidney, which reflexively secretes chemicals that promote salt and water retention, or edema. Premenstrual acceleration of this phenomenon is common.

SKIN COMPLAINTS

Some fibromyalgia patients have more than tender points under their skin. The skin itself is tender to touch. A manifestation of widespread allodynia, or heightened pain perception, this discomfort is present in more severe cases and is especially prevalent in patients taking steroids and in those who develop reflex sympathetic dystrophy (see Chapter 13).

There is no rash, per se, that is a unique feature of fibromyalgia. More patients than would be expected in the general population report dry skin, hair loss, itching, mouth sores, and easy bruisibility, although none of these complaints has yet been studied scientifically to determine if specific dermatologic problems are associated with fibromyalgia. Fibromyalgia patients also take more aspirin, ibuprofen, and other similar nonsteroidal antiinflammatory drugs, which can result in black-and-blue marks under the skin.

As discussed earlier, autonomic dysfunction produces changes under the skin that mimic Raynaud's phenomenon and cause *livedo reticularis,* a lace-like mottling of the skin that usually produces no symptoms (see Chapter 7). It's not uncommon for fibromyalgia patients to have a ruddy complexion or red palms along with this condition.

GENITOURINARY COMPLAINTS

A variety of fibromyalgia-related conditions to be reviewed in Chapter 13 are associated with symptoms such as aggravation of premenstrual pain, the sensation of needing to void all the time, painful intercourse, and vulvar tightness.

GASTROINTESTINAL COMPLAINTS

Significant problems relating to the gastrointestinal tract, present in one-third of fibromyalgia patients, are part of the *functional bowel spectrum,* which is discussed in detail in Chapter 13. Some of the major symptoms noted in this group of patients include diarrhea alternating with constipation, flatulence, distention, bloating, heartburn, stools with mucous, and diffuse abdominal pain.

ODDS AND ENDS: SMOKING AND VITAMIN D

Individuals with chronic back pain, fibromyalgia, and musculoskeletal pain are more likely to be smokers. Whether this is due to chronic coughing, those looking for alternative coping mechanisms, or a direct effect of tobacco on pain is unclear.

Vitamin D is a fat soluble vitamin responsible for the body's absorption of calcium and phosphorus. Sunlight is also a source, as are diet and supplements. Low vitamin D levels have long been associated with inflammatory and autoimmune disorders. Recently, several studies have documented that a statistically increased number of fibromyalgia patient have vitamin D insufficiency. Low vitamin D levels may be associated with musculoskeletal discomfort.

SUMMING UP

A surprisingly wide range of multisystemic symptoms and signs in healthy-appearing people can be a source of frustration and misunderstanding among patients, family members, and physicians. Many of these complaints are part of regional fibromyalgia syndromes, or *fibromyalgia-associated conditions,* which are reviewed in the next three chapters. Table 6.2 lists the frequency of the principal complaints among fibromyalgia patients.

FOR FURTHER READING

Almansa C, Wang B, Achem SR. Non cardiac chest pain and fibromyalgia. *Med Clin North Am.* 2010; *94*: 275–289.

Daniel D, Pirotta MV, Fibromyalgia—should we be testing and treating for vitamin D deficiency? *Aust Fam Physician.* 2011 Sep; *40*(9): 712–716.

Deoehar AA, Fischer RA, Blacker CVR, Woolf AD. Fluid retention syndrome and fibromyalgia. *Brit J Rheumatol 33*, 1994: 576–582.

Lee SS, Kim SH, Nah SS, *et al.* Smoking habits influence pain and function and psychiatric features in fibromyalgia. *Joint Bone Spine.* 2011 May; *78*(3): 259–265.

Part IV
THE CLINICAL SPECTRUM OF FIBROMYALGIA

Those who manage fibromyalgia respect its diversity of symptoms and signs. They appreciate and respect that it overlaps with other syndromes and disorders. Some of these conditions are, in truth, fibromyalgia masquerading under another name, and the very existence of others has been questioned. Local or regional forms of fibromyalgia add to the syndrome's complexity. This part will detail the manifestations that patients with these symptoms and signs experience and place them in the overall context of fibromyalgia syndrome.

12

What Are the Regional and Localized Forms of Fibromyalgia?

Physicians think they do a lot for a patient when they give his disease a name.

Immanuel Kant (1724–1804)

The definition of fibromyalgia includes widespread pain in all four quadrants (areas) of the body. What happens when you have fibromyalgia-like pain located in only one or two quadrants of the body? Limited forms of the syndrome have distinct features and terms used to describe them. *Myofascial pain syndrome* encompasses many regional pain conditions ranging from temporomandibular joint dysfunction in the jaw to a low back pain syndrome. The diagnosis of myofascial pain syndrome requires that at least one trigger point be present and that, when it is pressed, pain is referred to another site. This chapter will review regional myofascial pain, relate it to fibromyalgia pain pathways, and discuss its management and prognosis.

A BIT OF HISTORY: THE CONTRIBUTIONS OF PHYSICAL MEDICINE SPECIALISTS

Our current concepts of tender points, trigger points, and regional pain amplification were developed by two of the best-known physical medicine thinkers, Janet Travell and David Simons. Beginning in the early 1940s, Dr. Travell became well known as John F. Kennedy's physician, who nursed him back to health in the 1950s when back pain restricted his ability to walk. Later, she became Lyndon Johnson's White House physician. Travell and Simon's textbook on myofascial pain remains a classic and was updated by them as recently as 1992. Dr. Travell (who died in 1997 at the age of 95) and Dr. Simons formed close working relationships with rheumatologists, and their influence permeates every fibromyalgia study relating to tender points and regional pain.

Neurologists, neurosurgeons, and orthopedists diagnosed and treated localized muscle and nerve pain long before there were rheumatologists. At about the same time that rheumatologists were becoming recognized and organized into a certifiable subspecialty, an equally small group of doctors were organizing themselves into a specialty known as *physical medicine and rehabilitation.* These doctors (who call themselves *physiatrists*) do not perform surgery, are not internists or family physicians, and do not manage autoimmune diseases. They concern themselves with areas not addressed by rheumatologists such as stroke, cardiac, and spinal cord injury rehabilitation. Physical medicine doctors usually practice in a hospital or hospital-like environment and work closely on a daily basis with physical therapists, occupational therapists, speech therapists, social workers, psychologists, and other allied health professionals. They supervise most of the inpatient rehabilitation centers in the United States. Although they have never numbered more than a few thousand, physiatrists have developed important insights into regional fibromyalgia-like pain that are reviewed in this chapter.

WHAT CAUSES REGIONAL MYOFASCIAL PAIN?

Most regional myofascial discomfort is produced by trauma. Unlike fibromyalgia, in which nearly 50 inciting factors have been implicated, localized or regional myofascial pain syndrome is usually due to either a single traumatic event or repetitive injury.

Numerous factors contribute to myofascial problems. The term *myofascia* refers to both muscles (*myo-*) and the *fascia,* the thin layer of tissue covering, supporting, and separating muscles. Abnormal posture can produce local discomfort. For example, scoliosis may be associated with midback or scapular pain on one side. A patient who has had lower extremity orthopedic surgery and needs to walk with a cane or crutch for a few weeks and is not used to it may place abnormal stress on the back, hips, shoulder, or elbow, resulting in a temporary regional pain syndrome.

From a physiologic standpoint, most of the neurochemical pathways reviewed in Chapters 4–7 play a role in regional body syndromes. However, in regional myofascial pain, more emphasis is placed on sensitization of a primary nociceptor, a nerve that receives painful stimuli and transmits that information to the spinal cord. This results in secondary hyperalgesia (more pain than would normally be expected in an area), allodynia (an ordinarily painless stimulus that produces pain), and/or referred pain. Pain that occurs from stretching a muscle is due to reflex spasm secondary to altered peripheral nociception elsewhere. Prolonged shortening of a muscle increases pain, as does overuse in the form of a sustained muscle contraction. Sustained altered body mechanics results in sensitization of a primary nociceptor and subsequent regional hyperalgesia, allodynia, and referred pain. Tender points are common. These are hyperirritable loci found at musculotendinous junctions near nerves where mechanical forces cause microinjuries, whereby altered central nociception around them leads to enlarged receptor fields and referred pain. How does this happen? The signature feature is the trigger point, a tender, taut band of muscle that can be painful spontaneously or when stimulated. The active trigger point has identifiable physiologic changes. Levels of substance P, calcitonin gene related peptide, bradykinin, and assorted cytokines, are elevated, indicating a chemical inflammation all of which activate peripheral nociceptors. Trigger point milieu pH is low, consistent with hypoxia (lack of oxygen) and ischemia. Persistent, low-amplitude, high frequency electrical discharges that look like endplate potentials are characteristic. The taut band, chronically contracted, displays a sympathetic nervous system-modulated excessive endplate potential activity noise which produces a localized, non-propagated contraction. The net effect is an excess of acetylcholine at the motor end plate. Post-synaptic events in the muscle cell that promote prolonged contraction are those that increase the concentration of calcium, from the sarcoplasmic reticulum of the muscle through a dysfunction receptor in the calcium channel, by a second messenger system mediated by the sympathetic nervous system, or by mitochrondria and could result in persistent muscle fiber contraction.

Tender points play a major role in regional musculoskeletal pain. Tender points are hyperirritable loci found at muscle-tendon junctions near nerves where mechanical forces cause microinjuries. Researchers have found vasoconstriction in the skin above along with a slightly lower temperature, indicating that the ANS plays a role here. Local injury of tender points decreases the firing threshold of nerves as the stimulation of local nociceptors promotes the release of cytokines.

Referred pain relates to discomfort in areas that are near but not in the injured region or the affected tender points. Referred pain is produced by altered central nociception and enlarged receptor fields. Nociceptor input can be referred to another area served by receptors that converge in the spinothalamic tract. It can be very misleading. For instance, suppose that an area on the left side near your midcervical spine is extremely uncomfortable. The traumatic insult that led to this condition might be in the back of the shoulder, but pain is referred to this area near the spine. For therapists, focusing rehabilitation energies on areas of referred pain is not as rewarding as dealing with the primary, inciting biochemical problem. Figure 12.1 illustrates example of referred pain.

WHAT DOES A DOCTOR EXPECT TO SEE IN REGIONAL FORMS OF FIBROMYALGIA?

Patients with regional myofascial pain syndrome generally do not fulfill the ACR criteria for fibromyalgia. A distinct minority of patients with regional myofascial pain have systemic symptoms associated with fibromyalgia, such as fatigue, poor concentration, bloating, generalized weakness, and nonrestorative sleep. They tend to be slightly younger than most fibromyalgia patients and include more males. Pain occurs in an injured area long beyond its expected normal healing time and is chronic due to altered nociception or abnormal transmission of pain signals.

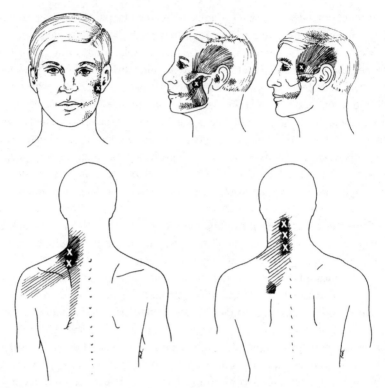

Fig. 12.1. *(top) TMJ dysfunction syndrome: Tender points (X) and referred pain areas. (bottom left) Upper back (trapezius) tender points (X) and areas of referred pain. (bottom right) Occipital (back of the neck) tender points (X) and referred pain areas.*

Myofascial pain syndrome can occur anywhere in the body, but more than 90% of these cases involve one of the following five regional combinations: neck and upper torso; temporomandibular joint (atypical facial pain, or TMJ); neck, arm, hand; low back, buttock, leg; and the chest area, including costochondritis. See Figure 12.1 for example.

EXAMPLES OF WELL-KNOWN SUBSETS OF REGIONAL MYOFASCIAL PAIN

Two of the best-known examples of regional myofascial pain involve jaw discomfort and repetitive strain disorder. Most TMJ patients consult ear, nose, or throat specialists, dentists, or orthopedists, as opposed to rheumatologists. In more serious cases, localized symptoms ultimately are connected to a systemic process such as fibromyalgia.

TMJ Dysfunction Syndrome

Dorothy began having trouble chewing meat, but this did not bother her since she was thinking of becoming a vegetarian. When she visited her sister's house and tried to play her niece's flute (something she had not done since high school), her left jaw felt as though it was being lanced by a sharp spear. Dorothy consulted her dentist, who found a very tight, tender TMJ. Dr. East sent her for imaging X-ray views of the TMJ, which were normal. She was diagnosed as having TMJ dysfunction syndrome. When Dorothy consulted her internist, Dr. Radford also noticed a lot of tightness and spasm on the left side of her neck and elicited a history of left-sided headaches in the back of her neck. Dorothy was started on ibuprofen, 600 mg three times a day, and was given jaw exercises and a muscle relaxant to take at night for a few weeks. A physical therapy referral was also given so that Dorothy could learn how to perform the exercises correctly, and a bite plate was fashioned for bedtime use. After two–three months, the TMJ symptoms eased. Dorothy now takes just ibuprofen occasionally.

Jaw pain is very uncomfortable and stems from many different sources. These include malocclusion, or an abnormal bite; arthritis of the joint (in rheumatoid arthritis and, to a less severe degree, in osteoarthritis); infection; bruxism, or teeth grinding; and traumatic injury. Myofascial pain from muscular spasm, with or without upper back and neck pain on the affected side, is a diagnosis of exclusion termed *temporomandibular joint dysfunction syndrome*. The pain stems from the same sources causing fibromyalgia and is amplified by anxiety, stress, or trauma, leading to unconscious jaw-closing movements. This regional form of fibromyalgia is diagnosed only after a dental evaluation and an ear, nose, and throat evaluation by a specialist, along with a special type of X-ray or imaging scan of the TMJ.

TMJ dysfunction syndrome afflicts approximately 10 million Americans; 70% are female. In a recent survey, 18% fulfilled the criteria for fibromyalgia and 75% of those with fibromyalgia had TMJ dysfunction. The temples, neck, and upper back can be affected. The TMJ dysfunction syndrome is treated with NSAIDs such as ibuprofen or naproxen, as well as moist heat, joint spacers (bite plates) worn at night, exercises, acupuncture and a technique known as *spray and stretch* (see Chapter 19). Occasionally, injecting the TMJ joint with a small amount of steroid and a local anesthetic such as xylocaine may be useful. Most general management features that are reviewed in Part VI may also be recommended or prescribed. Once the diagnosis of TMJ syndrome is made, expensive and unnecessary surgery should be avoided except in extreme cases and only after several expert opinions are obtained.

Repetitive Strain Syndrome

Over the last few years, Geoffrey Littlejohn and his associates in Australia have performed pioneering work on musculoskeletal problems observed in the workplace. With Australia's generous worker's compensation system and excellent data collection methodologies, his group helped nurture our current concepts of repetitive stress syndromes. A discipline known as *ergonomics,* which is a hybrid of kinesiology (the science or study of movement), engineering, and physics, has explored the science of human performance at work. Practitioners have developed information about what types of local stress individuals can sustain in a work environment over a period of time. For example, working at a computer all day or lifting shipping cartons onto a truck are forms of repetitive strain, as illustrated in Jared's case in Chapter 3. Many patients in the former category might complain of pain in the shoulder, with numbness and tingling in the hand. Anti-inflammatory medication, physical therapy, and even a local injection of an anesthetic, with or without corticosteroids, is only temporarily beneficial if the fundamental ergonomics of the workstation are not adapted to the patient's requirements.

Some of these considerations, along with disability issues, are reviewed in more detail in Part VII.

If repetitive strain syndrome is not adequately addressed and the patient continues to engage in an ergonomically unsatisfactory job environment, not only might disability and chronic regional pain be the consequence but full-blown fibromyalgia can evolve.

TREATMENT OF MYOFASCIAL PAIN SYNDROME

Myofascial pain syndrome is treated with a multidisciplinary approach that includes a variety of health care professionals such as physical therapy, occupational therapy, pain management, rheumatology, chiropractic, and physical medicine specialists among others. These treatments include:

- Physical medicine treatments such as heat, stretching, exercise, physical therapy
- Manual therapy such as myofascial release, trigger point therapy, and manipulation
- Spray and stretch involves cold modality followed by muscle stretching
- Trigger point injections with lidocaine with or without a small amount of steroid. Multiple injections may be helpful as well
- Medications include analgesics, anti-inflammatory regimens, muscle relaxants, anti-depressants, and anti-convulsants
- Supplements encompass vitamins, herbal preparations, and dietary foods among others

- Patient education optimizes body mechanics, introduces stress and anxiety reduction measures, and improves coping skills.

SUMMING UP

The outcome of regional pain syndromes is generally very good to excellent, usually much better than that of fibromyalgia. Delays in treatment, incorrect treatment, or continued injury to the affected region have adverse consequences that can allow fibromyalgia to develop. The management of regional myofascial syndromes is outlined in Part VII.

FOR FURTHER READING

Campbell SM. Regional myofascial pain syndromes. *Rheum Dis Clin North Am* 1989; *15*: 31–44.

Gerwin R. Myofascial pain syndrome: Here we are, where must we go? *J Musculoskeletal Pain* 2010; *18*: 329–346.

Hubbard J. Persistent muscular pain: Approaches to relieving trigger points. *J Musculoskeletal Pain 15*, 1998: 16–26.

Simmons DG. Clinical and etiologic update of myofascial pain from trigger points. *J Muscuolskeletal Pain 4*, 1996: 93–121.

13

What Conditions Are Associated with Fibromyalgia?

The fate of a nation has often depended upon the good or bad digestion of a prime minister.

Voltaire (1694–1778)

The perception of fibromyalgia as a distinct syndrome is relatively new. As recounted in Chapter 1, healers and sufferers have struggled to define what people have and how they feel with regard to widespread pain and fatigue complaints since the time of Job. Throughout this century, patients with fibromyalgia-like complaints have been diagnosed by physicians as having all types of conditions, syndromes, and diseases. Many of these overlap with fibromyalgia and this chapter focuses on the most important ones.

CHRONIC FATIGUE SYNDROME

Friends always thought Kathy was an overachiever. They marveled that she could be an exemplary mother devoted to her two children and hold down a high-powered executive position while still finding time to run the church auxiliary and play tennis six hours a week. When she missed work for three days with a temperature of 102°F, a sore throat, cough, and swollen neck glands, nobody anticipated what followed. Although she returned to work the next week, it was clear that something had changed. Kathy was too tired to play tennis and started going to bed early. She began having difficulty thinking clearly and complained to her doctor about a "fog" in her brain. When the weather changed, Kathy reported being more stiff and achy. Ultimately, Kathy was diagnosed as having a postinfectious fatigue syndrome. She took a leave of absence from her job, but the company hired her as a consultant to help out with specific projects, which allowed her to work at a more leisurely pace. After 18 months, she returned to her job. Kathy seemed to be herself but was working at about 80% of her previous level.

The codification and "legitimization" of fibromyalgia with statistically validated criteria has paralleled similar initiatives concerning *chronic fatigue syndrome* (CFS). Chapter 1 recounted some of the earlier insights and efforts.

An acute infection is often characterized by fever, swollen glands, and either a cold/bronchitis, a stomach/intestinal condition, or an aching/debilitating presentation. As the body fights infection and makes antibodies against microbes, acute symptoms and signs start to disappear and most of the time patients feel much better. However, a variety of organisms can stimulate the production of cytokines (discussed in Chapter 6) and other chemicals, which prolong fatigue and aching and may be associated with cognitive impairment, malaise, pain amplification, and sleeping difficulties.

How the Centers for Disease Control Drew Up Criteria for CFS

Between 1930 and 1980, it was known that some patients recovering from infectious diseases such as polio, mononucleosis, and brucellosis had a prolonged convalescence and persistent systemic symptoms. By the early 1980s, a herpes virus known as Epstein-Barr virus joined the group (mononucleosis is also a herpes virus). For unknown reasons, it tended to afflict upwardly mobile young people, and the press tagged Epstein-Barr virus as a "yuppie flu disease." Epstein-Barr virus antibodies could easily be tested for, and its postviral fatigue complaints were treated symptomatically and waited out.

However, the "Epstein-Barr syndrome" epidemic turned out not to happen. The National Institutes of Health, United States Centers for Disease Control and Prevention (CDC), and other centers showed that over half of the U.S. population has evidence of exposure to Epstein-Barr virus in their blood, and standard antiviral therapy for herpes was not beneficial in these patients. Some Epstein-Barr patients had significant primary psychiatric problems, and numerous other organisms (e.g., bacteria, viruses, fungi, parasites) were shown to cause postinfectious fatigue syndromes. Chronic Epstein-Barr virus fatigue syndrome did exist, but it was overdiagnosed and in fact is relatively rare.

In 1984, I suggested in a medical journal article that fatigue syndromes and fibromyalgia could be one and the same. This hunch was documented when three world-renowned experts at Boston University tried an experiment. Drs. Anthony Komaroff and Dedra Buchwald, the most preeminent Epstein-Barr/chronic fatigue specialists in the United States at the time, had their clinic patients see a highly respected fibromyalgia expert, Dr. Donald Goldenberg. When Dr. Goldenberg's patients were sent to the Komaroff-Buchwald clinic, these doctors soon realized that the majority of their patients had both CFS and fibromyalgia.

The CDC devised statistically validated criteria for CFS in 1988, which were updated in 1994 (Table 13.1). The current definition of CFS requires unexplained,

Table 13.1. *The CDC Revised Criteria for CFS (1994)*

1. Chronic fatigue of unknown cause that persists or returns for more than 6 months, resulting in a substantial reduction in occupational, educational, social, or personal activities.
2. The presence of 4 or more of the following symptoms concurrently for more than 6 months:
   a. Sore throat
   b. Tender cervical or axillary lymph glands
   c. Muscle pain
   d. Multijoint pain
   e. New headaches
   f. Unrefreshing sleep
   g. Postexertion malaise
   h. Cognitive dysfunction

clinically evaluated fatigue of new or definite onset lasting for at least six months and not relieved with rest that substantially impairs performance. New onset of four of the following eight factors must also be present: cognitive impairment, sore throat, tender cervical or axillary lymph nodes, muscle aches, joint aches, headache, sleep disorder, and malaise after exertion lasting longer than one day. By definition, patients with primary psychiatric disorders cannot have CFS. Using the aforementioned criteria, the prevalence of CFS in the United States is somewhere between 100,000 and 300,000, with several hundred thousand other persons having unexplained chronic fatigue without CFS. According to a studies conducted in the United States and Great Britain, 4% of the population complained of chronic fatigue. If coexisting psychiatric (especially stress, childhood trauma, emotional instability) and medical disorders (especially anemia, hypothyroidism, hepatitis C and lupus) were excluded, 0.1–0.5% of the population fulfilled criteria for CFS.

Sometimes, CFS is referred to as *chronic fatigue immune dysfunction syndrome* (CFIDS). The authors prefer the term CFS since immune dysfunction is neither a proven nor prominent feature of the syndrome. Surprisingly little has been published in chronic fatigue syndrome since 2000. Advocates of it as a diagnostic entity feel that inflammation, immune system activation, autonomic dysfunction, impaired functioning in the HPA axis, and neuroendocrine dysregulation alone or in combination are root causes of fatigue. Other practitioners state that it is no different than fibromyalgia. Several causative factors such as the XMRV virus have been discredited.

CFS and Fibromyalgia: Similarities and Differences

The majority of patients diagnosed with CFS in the United States are between the ages of 20 and 50, female, and Caucasian. Comparative surveys show that 20–70% of fibromyalgia patients have CFS, and 35–70% of those with CFS have fibromyalgia. CFS patients have greater elevations of antiviral antibodies than is observed in fibromyalgia. Whereas only a minority of fibromyalgia patients complain of a sore throat, show evidence of swollen glands or fevers, and have onset after a flu-like illness, these features are found in most CFS patients (Table 13.2). Although one well-regarded theory suggests that CFS is manifested after exposure to repeated viral infections in the setting of an overactive immune state, immune blood testing is inconsistent, contradictory, expensive, and does not change our treatment.

Autonomic dysfunction is common in CFS. This leads to low blood pressure in many of these patients, which is manifested clinically as *neurally mediated hypotension,* that aggravates fatigue. Here sympathetic activity produces a low resting volume. This excessive pooling of blood on dependent vessels produces an excessive loss of plasma when standing up. Cognitive impairment has also been documented with hypoperfusion on SPECT scanning, with the brain intermittently not getting enough oxygen.

THE FUNCTIONAL BOWEL SPECTRUM

Lilly always had a sensitive stomach, and whenever she was stressed it seemed that things ran right through her. As the vice president of a garment manufacturing company on the West Coast, she traveled to Asia at least once a month. Over time, Lilly developed frequent bouts of diarrhea alternating with constipation. She would be very gaseous, and her abdomen became intermittently distended. Lilly was sure she had picked up a parasite, and her internist, after obtaining normal blood and stool tests, referred her to a gastroenterologist. Dr. Sharp had also been aware of her complaints of mild aching and fatigue. He performed a colonoscopy and an endoscopy (procedures that allow a doctor to view the colon, esophagus, and stomach) and took biopsy specimens and cultures. Nothing was found. Lilly was started on hyoscyamine (Levsin), a drug that reduces intestinal muscle spasms and a higher-fiber diet, with substantial relief. She was diagnosed as

Table 13.2. *Comparisons of Fibromyalgia and CFS*

Parameter	Fibromyalgia (%)	Chronic fatigue syndrome (%)
Female sex	90	80
Muscle aches	99	80
Joint aches	99	75
Fatigue	90	99
Poor sleep	80	50
Complaints of fever	28	75
Complaints of swollen glands	33	80
Postexertional fatigue	80	80
Sudden or acute onset	55	70
Headaches	60	85
Cognitive dysfunction	20	65

having irritable bowel syndrome and returned to her primary care provider, who spent time with her working on lifestyle and dietary modifications.

The diagnosis a patient receives is usually influenced by the physician's background and training. For example, more than half of the internal medicine specialists in the United States have subspecialty training. Therefore, a patient who consults three different internists with training in infectious disease, rheumatology, or gastroenterology might be given a diagnosis of CFS, fibromyalgia, or functional bowel disease, respectively.

Over the last decade, functional bowel disease has become a spectrum of gastroenterologic disorders with a common link of *visceral hyperalgesia*, or increased pain sensitivity in the internal structures. Identified by a variety of terms including *spastic colitis, irritable colon, diffuse abdominal pain*,

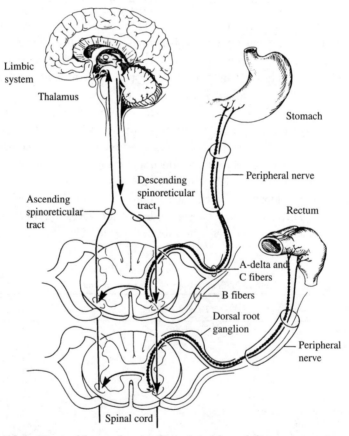

Fig. 13.1. *Visceral hyperalgesia. Functional bowel disease symptoms are thought to result from the amplification of parasympathetic nervous system B-fiber signals.*

noncardiac chest pain, and *nonulcer dyspepsia,* this spectrum was once primarily thought to be a motility, or movement, disorder. In fact, it has turned out to be a pain amplification disorder. Initiated by inciting factors that cause peripheral or visceral pain fibers and the parasympathetic nervous system to promote primary and secondary hyperalgesia with central sensitization, the functional bowel spectrum substantially overlaps with fibromyalgia. Patients report increased perception of stomach movements and distension. This lower sensory threshold leads to abdominal pain and discomfort. Recent evidence suggests that a neuropeptide found in the limbic system of the brain and the gut, cholecystokinin, produces abdominal or intestinal muscle spasms. Figure 13.1 illustrates these pathways.

Functional bowel complaints are the most common reason for referral to a gastroenterologist. As with fibromyalgia, 2% of the U.S. population fulfill the criteria for functional bowel disease, but as many as 20% may have it at some point. In the United States, 70% are female, and it costs $8 billion a year to diagnose and treat it. Patients report abdominal distention, bloating, pain relief

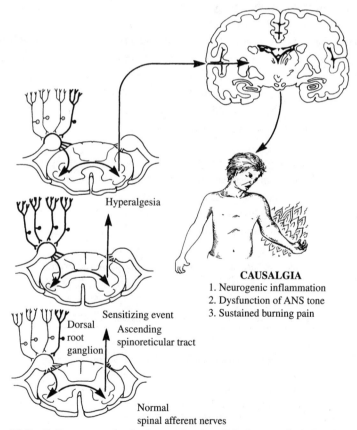

Fig. 13.2. *Reflex sympathetic dystrophy. Amplified musculoskeletal pain is complicated by ANS reactions that lead to severe burning, pain, and swelling.*

Table 13.3. *Summary of Definitions for Functional Bowel Syndrome Based on the Rome and Manning Criteria*

At least 3 months of continuous and recurrent symptoms and signs of the following:
1. Abdominal pain and discomfort relieved with defecation or associated with change in stool consistency
2. Two of the following five factors listed below on at least 25% of daily occasions: mucous in stool, bloating/distension, altered stool frequency (more than 3 a day or less than 3 a week), altered stool passage, altered stool form.
Incomplete sense of evacuation

with bowel movements, more frequent and loose stools with the onset of pain, frequent mucus in bowel movements, a sensation of incomplete evacuation, flatulence, and cramping. Some doctors believe that food allergies or medication sensitivity aggravate the syndrome. The criteria for diagnosing functional bowel disease are listed in Table 13.3.

Fibromyalgia complaints extend beyond the small intestine or colon. For example, sensitization of different parts of the spinal cord and referred pain can lead to persistent upper abdominal nonulcer pain and chest pains. Recent studies suggest that approximately 40% of patients with functional bowel disease fulfill the criteria for fibromyalgia and vice versa. Functional bowel disease affects a type of muscle known as *involuntary*, or *smooth*, muscle. By contrast, fibromyalgia tender points overlie voluntary, striated, or skeletal muscle.

In the last decade, symptoms in the functional bowel spectrum have been shown to be part of a variety of other associated pathophysiologic, inflammatory, and infectious components. These include (See Table 13.4):

- SIBO, or small intestinal bacterial overgrowth. Our group has correlated increased intestinal permeability (degree of leakiness of the intestinal epithelial layer to luminal products) with FM. Measured by a hydrogen breath test and associated with abnormal motility studies, this distention and bloating responds to broad spectrum antibiotics, particularly rifaximin and neomycin at least temporarily as well as probiotics.
- Celiac disease is an autoimmune disorder characterized by sensitivity to gluten or wheat products. It can be diagnosed by blood testing for

Table 13.4. *The Spectrum of Functional Gastrointestinal Disorders*

- Esophageal—functional chest pain, heartburn, dysphagia
- Gastroduodenal—Dyspepsia (functional, ulcer-like, dysmotility-like), aerophagia (swallowing air), functional vomiting, *helicobacter pylori*
- Bowel—irritable bowel syndrome (IBS), functional abdominal bloating, narcotic bowel syndrome, constipation, or diarrhea. Celiac disease, lymphocytic colitis, ulcerative colitis, Crohn's disease, *C. Difficile, campylobacter jejuni*
- Functional abdominal pain related to psychosocial stressors
- Functional biliary tract disorders—gallbladder or sphincter of Oddi dysfunction
- Anorectal—anorectal pain, fecal incontinence, proctalgia fugax, pelvic floor dyssynergia

antibodies or a bowel biopsy. Statistically associated with fibromyalgia, celiac disease responds to dietary modifications.

- Lymphocytic colitis and inflammatory bowel disease represent the stimulation of immunocompetent cells and are associated with bacterial overgrowth.
- Bacterial infections of the gut such as *camplylobacter jejuni, Yersinia enterocolitica* in the intestine or *helicobacter pylori*, which causes gastric ulcers. All are managed with antibiotic regimens.
- Narcotic bowel syndrome/laxative abuse in patients taking large amounts of analgesic medications paralyzes the bowel with or without requirements to use regular laxatives. This creates motility issues and can be diagnosed by the presence of "melanosis coli" at colonoscopy. It is treated by narcotic detoxification and psychopathologic interventions.

AUTOIMMUNE DISEASES

Ronna developed stiffness and aching in her hands and feet. At age 30, when Dr. Dale evaluated her, she looked great and the examination of her hands and feet was normal. Dr. Dale performed blood tests that showed slight anemia, a low white blood cell count, and a slightly elevated sedimentation rate (a blood test for inflammation). Dr. Dale told Ronna that her anemia was due to heavy periods and placed her on iron. Her low white blood cell count and elevated sedimentation rate could be explained by a cold she had two weeks before, and he told her to come back in six months. Ronna began developing pain in her upper back and neck area and started having muscle spasms. Six months later she had obvious swelling in her wrists and was markedly anemic; her white blood cell count was very low and her sedimentation rate quite elevated. Dr. Dale did further testing that showed she had systemic lupus erythematosus, an autoimmune disease, on the basis of positive antinuclear antibody (ANA) and anti-DNA tests. He explained to her that her fibromyalgia-like complaints represented her body's reaction to the untreated inflammation of lupus.

Anywhere from 10–30% of patients with primary Sjogren's, systemic lupus erythematosus, Hashimoto's thyroiditis, or rheumatoid arthritis also have FM. The reasons include untreated or undertreated inflammation (leading to central sensitization or activation of other central pain amplification mechanisms), hyperesthesia produced by steroids, or steroid withdrawal syndromes. Patients with autoimmune conditions commonly have disease related psychosocial distress and difficulty coping, which can produce or aggravate FM. It can be difficult to distinguish FM from autoimmune complaints; the presence of acute phase reactants supports the latter. Patients with FM are also often misdiagnosed as having an autoimmune disorder.

LYME DISEASE

As a high school senior, Natalie was selected to attend a regional youth retreat in rural Connecticut. The mosquitoes found her very attractive, and she noticed a quarter-sized, expanding red rash on her left leg a week after she returned to Manhattan. Nevertheless, she felt well and the spot faded. Several weeks later, Natalie developed flu-like symptoms and complained of muscle and joint aches. The results of the blood tests performed by her physician, Dr. Garth, strongly suggested Lyme disease, and he gave her antibiotics in high doses for several weeks. Except for some fluid in her right knee that had to be drained, Natalie seemed to improve overall, but she never felt quite the same. She noticed increased sensitivity to changes in the weather and on being touched, difficulty getting a good night's sleep, and increased anxiety. Dr. Garth diagnosed her condition as post-Lyme fibromyalgia. Natalie did not need additional antibiotics and was prescribed Sinequan drops at bedtime, which she took regularly for a few months and now uses only occasionally.

Since the mid-1970s, physicians have known that a deer-borne tick, *Ixodes dammini,* can infect people with a spirochete bacterium known as *Borrelia burg-dorferi.* The disease was named for the area around Lyme, Connecticut, where it was first described; 90% of all cases are reported in the New England and mid-Atlantic regions.

Lyme disease is a complex malady. It presents in three stages. About one-third of tick bites are followed within a month by a distinct rash known as *erythema chronicum migrans.* Several weeks later, patients develop a generalized flu-like condition that may include joint swelling, muscle and joint aches, headache, sore throat, cough, fever, and swollen glands. If they are not treated with antibiotics (and infrequently if they have been treated), about 10% of the original group go on to a third stage in which potentially serious heart or nervous system involvement can develop.

What does fibromyalgia have to do with Lyme disease? First, a postinfectious fatigue/fibromyalgia syndrome ultimately afflicts a minority of Lyme disease patients. Second, many people who were told they had Lyme disease in fact had fibromyalgia. The reasoning is similar to what has been related about the Epstein-Barr virus. Some blood tests for Lyme disease are not very reliable for diagnosing the disease, and many patients who consult a doctor for fibromyalgia-like symptoms have evidence of prior exposure to the Lyme disease-inducing spirochete bacterium. Does this simply represent being in an endemic area where many residents have been exposed, or is the condition actually a postinfectious Lyme fibromyalgia? There is an important reason to try to determine this. Patients who have evidence of Lyme disease should receive a course of antibiotics in order to prevent the more serious third stage of the disease. However, this expensive and time-consuming therapy is rarely necessary. If a primary care physician is not sure what to do, rheumatology or infectious disease specialty evaluations may be useful.

COMPLEX REGIONAL PAIN SYNDROME (REFLEX SYMPATHETIC DYSTROPHY; CRPS, RSD)

It was a freak accident. Olivia was riding in a golf cart with her husband when he swerved to avoid a large rock and the cart overturned. She dislocated her left shoulder and underwent emergency surgery to repair it. Even though the repair was technically perfect, Dr. Bryan was concerned when her left hand swelled, the left shoulder remained immobile, and Olivia's excruciating pain persisted. A few days later, her right hand became swollen even though that side had not been injured. Dr. Bryan diagnosed her with reflex sympathetic dystrophy, injected her left shoulder with cortisone, and initiated a vigorous physical therapy program for her frozen shoulder. High doses of prednisone (a steroid) were also prescribed for ten days. Despite this therapy, Olivia's shoulder had to be manipulated under anesthesia so that she could move it. Although the swelling improved over the following months, Olivia's burning, tingling, and generalized musculoskeletal discomfort were intense. Dr. Bryan referred her to a pain management center, which used several simultaneous modalities, including pamidronate. Olivia's condition is slowly improving.

Reflex sympathetic dystrophy (RSD) can be induced by trauma, surgery, or certain drugs, or may occur spontaneously. A patient initially notices burning, tingling, and throbbing, sensitivity to touch or cold, and swelling of an arm or leg. A thorough examination usually demonstrates that both sides of the body are involved, although one side is more swollen than the other. The skin may be red or mottled. The affected extremity is painful to the touch and difficult to move. At first, a doctor may suspect a rheumatoid-like inflammatory arthritis. The swelling represents a form of neurogenic inflammation (see Chapter 7). In the second phase of CRPS (complex regional pain syndrome; see below), the swelling becomes brawny and thicker, with pigment changes three to six months later. The numbness, burning, and tingling persist. After one or two years, muscle atrophy and wasting are evident in the affected limb, affected bones become osteoporotic (termed *Sudeck's atrophy*), and range of motion may be decreased. The swelling disappears, but a chronic pain syndrome with generalized fibromyalgia develops. A milder, regional CRPS known as *shoulder-hand syndrome* is associated with a frozen or immobile shoulder.

CRPS/RSD is a form of sympathetically mediated pain. Officially designated as a "complex regional pain syndrome," it afflicts one person in 5,000. Occurring when peripheral sensory receptors are oversensitized or outgoing sympathetic impulses are short-circuited to incoming sensory fibers, RSD can be a type of *causalgia,* consisting of sustained burning pain with allodynia, increased reaction to a stimulus, and dysfunction of autonomically mediated blood vessel tone. In RSD, chronic nociceptive stimulation produces sympathetic nervous system reactions (illustrated in Figure 13.2). This painful condition is very frustrating and difficult to treat. RSD probably represents 1–2% of fibromyalgia patients in a community rheumatology practice (Table 13.5).

In its early phase, RSD should be managed aggressively with short courses of high-dose corticosteroids, vigorous mobilization, and physical therapy. Our group uses a bisphosphonate, pamidronate, intravenously, every 3 months. Once RSD has entered the second stage, some of its chronic features may be irreversible. Although the approaches used to treat fibromyalgia discussed in Part VI are useful, two additional aspects of RSD therapy need time and careful consideration. First, prolonged, aggressive physical therapy is helpful. Preferably, this should be prescribed in consultation with a physical medicine and rehabilitation specialist or orthopedist. Local steroid injections and sympathetic nervous system blockade are frequently helpful. Second, RSD patients may require narcotic pain medication in order to make it through the day, and a pain management consultation with follow-up may be advisable.

RSD patients are probably in more pain for longer periods of time than patients with most other rheumatic diseases. Once an RSD patient enters the second phase of the disease, a multidisciplinary approach is optimal: consultants from various specialties who communicate regularly to coordinate care provide the highest level of comfort and the best outcome for this unfortunate group of people.

PREMENSTRUAL SYNDROME AND DYSMENORRHEA

Naomi had a tendency to be stiff, achy, and tired. All of her blood tests were normal, and she was diagnosed as having fibromyalgia on the basis of her history and tender points on examination. Most of the time the condition

Table 13.5. *Budapest 2004 Revision of International Association for the Study of Pain Criteria for CRPS*

The presence of an initiating noxious event or a cause of immobilization

Continuing pain, allodynia, or hyperalgesia in which the pain is disproportionate to any known inciting event

Evidence at some time of edema, changes in skin blood flow, or abnormal sudomotor activity in the region of pain (can be a sign or symptom) <One in 3 or more of 4 categories as a symptom and one in 2 or more categories as a sign>

Diagnosis is excluded by the existence of other conditions that would otherwise account for the degree of pain and dysfunction

---

Adapted from: Harden R, Bruehl S, Diagnostic criteria: The statistical derivation of the Four Criterion Facors. In Wilson PR, CRPS: Current Diagnosis and Therapy, Progress in Pain Research and Management, 2005; 3: 45–58, IASP Press, Seattle, WA was mild and required no treatment. However, the symptoms greatly worsened a few days before her period started. Naomi became very irritable and difficult to talk to. She once failed a final exam in history, even though her mastery of the material was obvious, because of inability to concentrate. Naomi was concerned that she could lose her after-school sales job due to the mood swings related to *premenstrual syndrome* (PMS) that disturbed her co-workers and customers. Dr. Tash successfully treated Naomi with a combination regimen of ibuprofen and diuretics taken for three days every month premenstrually along with a muscle relaxant in the evening.

The release of hormones, prostaglandins, and other chemicals along with serotonin dysfunction prior to the onset of menses can cause fluid retention, a sense of bloating, alterations in mood and behavior, and occasionally painful periods (dysmenorrhea). While most women experience these cyclical alterations, 3–10% of American women have severe physical and psychological symptoms that interfere with their ability to function. They complain of irritability, tension, headache, backache, breast tenderness, depression, lack of energy, difficulty concentrating, a sleep disorder, and feeling "out of control." About 70% of women with fibromyalgia experience flares premenstrually, and the prevalence of fibromyalgia among those with more severe dysmenorrhea is increased. In addition to managing fibromyalgia, treating doctors frequently add an ibuprofen or naproxen-containing anti-inflammatory agent to be taken a few days just before the onset of menstruation. Other women report relief when they take a mild diuretic (water pill) for these few days as well.

CHRONIC PELVIC PAIN

As visceral structures, the urethra, bladder neck, vagina, prostate and rectum are attached to striated, or voluntary muscles. Visceral receptors are usually fairly silent. When abnormally activated, they can cause chronic pelvic pain.

Irritable Bladder, or Female Urethral Syndrome

Almost every hour Sherrie had to urinate, regardless of attempts at control. Sherrie seemed to have many bladder infections that never responded fully to antibiotics, although she always felt better while being treated. She often felt an intense, sudden urge to void, even though only dribbling occurred. Finally, her family physician referred Sherrie to a urologist. Dr. Stern obtained negative urine cultures. An X-ray known as an intravenous pyelogram (IVP) failed to demonstrate structural abnormalities in the kidney, ureter, or bladder. Dr. Stern performed cystoscopy (examining the bladder through a telescope inserted into the urethra) and found no inflammation, polyps, or tumors. There were no strictures in the urethra. Sherrie visited her family doctor a few weeks later because of tension headaches and muscle aches. Dr. Jones thought these symptoms were from a myofascial source. He prescribed cyclobenzaprine (Flexeril) at night, which, incidentally, greatly diminished her urge to void. At her next visit to Dr. Stern, he informed Sherrie that she was suffering from female urethral syndrome and added tolterodine (Detrol) to take during the day.

Among young women, urinary tract infections are extremely common. All too often, in order to make it convenient for the doctor and the patient, antibiotics are prescribed by telephone for symptoms and signs of burning with voiding, blood in the urine, or frequent urination. In an ideal world, antibiotics should be prescribed after a urine culture is obtained, and the prescription might be altered 48 to 72 hours later when the infecting organism has been grown and identified. Some patients have recurrent infections, and still others are on chronic antibiotic prophylactic therapy.

Within this population, a subgroup of young women fall through the cracks. They complain of intense pain with urination, and the urinalysis may show a few pus cells or red blood cells. The urine cultures are usually negative, and mechanical problems such as a urethral stricture or neurogenic bladder are not present. Sometimes the pain seems to lessen with an antibiotic, although this is usually because doctors frequently add anesthetic medicines (e.g., phenazopyridine [Pyridium]) to the antibiotic, which diminishes discomfort while voiding. These patients have *female urethral syndrome,* which our group was the first to associate with fibromyalgia. Representing spasm of the muscles around the urethra, an irritable bladder is found in 10–15% of fibromyalgia patients. Its management consists of reassurance, avoiding antibiotics, phenazopyridine hydrochlonde [Pyridium] (a urinary anesthetic), and antispasmodics (e.g., known as alpha blockers). We have found that when muscle relaxants such as diazepam (Valium) or cyclobenzaprine (Flexeril) are taken for a few nights, urethral spasm usually abates for periods ranging from days to months.

Interstitial Cystitis

Interstitial cystitis could be considered a controversial condition because of its lack of a clear-cut definition. Classic interstitial cystitis is defined as bladder and pelvic pain, frequency, and urinary urgency in a patient with negative urine cultures. Associated with voiding hesitancy, it worsens with menses and menopause. Cystoscopy reveals inflammation, blood, and frequently scarring when biopsy samples are viewed under the microscope. The bladder muscle wall can be thick and vascular with superficial ulcerations, but the lining mucosa is friable and thin. Classic interstitial cystitis is seen in autoimmune diseases (especially lupus), after radiation therapy, and in patients who had chronic bladder infections in the past.

Unfortunately, some practitioners (particularly non-urologists) term what we call female urethral syndrome (see Chapter 13) interstitial cystitis; others use the term loosely on the basis of the above-listed symptoms without cystoscopic confirmation. Recent studies have shown that a type of white blood cell known as a *mast cell* is present in large numbers at the nerve endings in interstitial cystitis patients. The bladder wall also has high levels of substance P. An increased percentage of patients who fall into the categories listed in this paragraph have fibromyalgia.

Vulvodynia and Vaginismus

Paulette was 11 when her stepfather molested her after drinking heavily. She was very frightened and did not tell anyone. As a young adult, her dating experiences were characterized by perfunctory, unenjoyed sex and difficulty forming close relationships. With time, her vaginal muscles tightened so much that penetration was impossible, and her vulvar area always hurt. Paulette's gynecologist could not find any structural abnormalities, tumors, or infection. Paulette never discussed these complaints with her internist, who had already diagnosed her with fibromyalgia on the basis of headaches, difficulty sleeping, aching, and fatigue. When her stepfather developed terminal cirrhosis of the liver, Paulette's fears and anxiety increased. She met with her internist, told her the whole story, and was referred for counseling. As a consequence, Paulette finally told her mother and sister what had happened. Her vulvar pain and vaginal tightness decreased, as did her fibromyalgia. She finally confronted her stepfather. Even though he denied everything, Paulette was finally able to obtain closure and get on with her life.

Seen in less than 5% of fibromyalgia patients, a small group of FM patients describe intense female genital tract discomfort, painful vulva without infection (*vulvodynia*), and/or involuntary spasm of the vaginal muscles when intercourse is attempted (*vaginismus*) with a normal gynecologic exam. Also known as "chronic pelvic congestion," this phenomenon comprises 2% of all gynecology visits in the United States. These complaints are statistically associated with irritable bladder complaints. The patient's psychosocial background may include a combination of behaviors or experiences including abuse, domestic violence, a family history of alcoholism, a rape experience, traumatic toilet training, abnormal bowel habits, dance training, pelvic trauma, pelvic inflammatory disease, and guilt surrounding sexual feelings. Repetitive minor trauma or straining at dance, gymnastics, and bicycling or certain other vigorous exercises also play a role. Treatments include counseling, anxiety reduction measures, psychotropic medications, sex therapy, botox injections, and pelvic floor musculature biofeedback. A small number of males develop a similar syndrome known as chronic prostatitis.

STEROID, HEROIN, ALCOHOL, OR COCAINE WITHDRAWAL

Ursula experienced a lot of aching in her hands and feet. At age 23, she was too young to develop arthritis. Dr. Abel could not find anything on examination and told Ursula to take Advil (an over-the-counter aspirin-like anti-inflammatory drug) when she felt pain. One month later, her knuckles began to swell, and upper back and lower buttock pain developed. Dr. Abel diagnosed her with early rheumatoid arthritis on the basis of Ursula's examination and the presence of rheumatoid factor in her blood. He also found myofascial tender areas in her upper and lower back regions that he explained would disappear with treatment. He was absolutely correct. Ursula took methotrexate, and her rheumatoid arthritis and fibromyalgia pains went away. After six months, however, blood test abnormalities forced Dr. Abel to stop the methotrexate and substitute low doses of prednisone (a steroid). When Ursula's rheumatoid arthritis continued to be stable, he decreased the dose of prednisone from 10 to 5 mg a day. Four days later, Ursula's myofascial tender points became unbearable but her rheumatoid arthritis stayed quiet. Dr. Abel prescribed amitriptyline (Elavil) for a few nights until her steroid-withdrawal fibromyalgia resolved.

Corticosteroids are prescribed for a variety of inflammatory and allergic conditions ranging from asthma, ulcerative colitis, and sinus irritation to rheumatoid arthritis and lupus, and along with chemotherapy for certain malignancies. When steroids are taken for more than a few weeks, the skin becomes very sensitive to touch or pressure. It also becomes sensitive to small alterations in steroid doses. For example, if a patient is taking 15 mg of prednisone and the dose is reduced to 10 mg, the decrease in dose can produce a *steroid withdrawal fibromyalgia.* This is not classical fibromyalgia because if the dose stays at 10 mg, most of the fibromyalgia-like pain and spasm disappear within a few weeks. Long-term steroid administration is associated with secondary fibromyalgia by causing increased skin and soft tissue sensitivity.

Acute, transient circumstances in which a temporary fibromyalgia-like situation occurs are also found in patients withdrawing from alcohol, heroin, or cocaine.

RESTLESS LEGS SYNDROME (SEE CHAPTER 10)

Tension Headache Syndrome, Mitral Valve Prolapse, and Others

Headaches are a common feature of fibromyalgia. Detailed histories indicate that many patients who seek neurologic consultation for tension headaches turn out to have fibromyalgia symptoms and signs. We discussed tension headaches

Table 13.6. *Fibromyalgia-associated Conditions*

Condition	% who have fibromyalgia	% with fibromyalgia who have associated conditions
Chronic fatigue syndrome	50	50
Functional bowel	20	40
Autoimmune disease	10	2
Lyme disease	30	2
Reflex dystrophy	100	5
Premenstrual syndrome	10	50
Female urethral syndrome	10	12
Vulvodynia, vaginismus	50	5
Mitral valve prolapse	10	20
Tension headache	20	53
TMJ dysfunction	18	75
U.S.population	2	—

in Chapter 10 and mitral valve prolapse in Chapter 11. Other syndromes associated with fibromyalgia include chronic hyperventilation, increased awareness of cardiac activity (palpitation sensations without mitral valve prolapse or cardiac abnormality) and globus hystericus (where patients continually complain of a lump in their throat).

SUMMING UP

Pain amplification, widespread pain, and systemic symptoms are not unique to fibromyalgia; variants of these three symptoms are found in many other conditions. Some conditions overlap with fibromyalgia to varying degrees and are managed with similar treatment approaches. Table 13.6 summarizes some of the relationships between fibromyalgia-associated conditions.

FOR FURTHER READING

Anothaisintawee T, Attia J, Nickel JC, *et al.* Management of chronic prostatitis/chronic pelvic pain syndrome. *JAMA* 2011; *305*: 78–86.

Chang L. The association of functional gastrointestinal disorders and fibromyalgia. *Eur J Surg* supp *583*, 1998: 32–36.

Clauw DJ, Schmidt M, Radulovic D, *et al.* The relationship between fibromyalgia and interstitial cystitis. *J Psychiat Res 31*, 1997: 125–131.

Dinerman H, Steere AC. Lyme disease associated with fibromyalgia. *Ann Intern Med 117*, 1992: 281–285.

Goebel A, Buhner S, Schedel R, *et al.* Altered intestinal permeability in patients with primary fibromyalgia and in patients with complex regional pain syndrome. *Rheumatology* 2008; *47*: 1223–1227.

Jones JF, Lin JM, Maloney EM, *et al*. An evaluation of exclusionary medical/psychiatric conditions in the definition of chronic fatigue syndrome. *BMC Med* 2009; 7:57.

Klimas NG, Broderick G, Fletcher MA. Biomarkers for chronic fatigue. *Brain Behav Immun* 2012; *26*: 1202–1210.

Kurland JE, Coyle WJ, Winkler A, Zable E. Prevalence of irritable bowel syndrome and depression in fibromyalgia. *Dig Dis Sci 51*, 2006; 454–460.

MacDonald KL, Osterholm MT, Le Dell KH, Sceuck CH, Chao CC, Persing DH, Johnson RC, Barker JM, Peterson PK. A case-control study to assess possible triggers and cofactors in chronic fatigue syndrome. *Amer J Med 100*, 1996: 548–554.

Moskowitz P. An overview of CRPS. *Practical Pain Management* 2010; Jan/Feb pp. 50–57.

Nickel JC, Tripp DA, Pontari M, *et al*. Interstitial cystitis/painful bladder syndrome and associated medical conditions with an emphasis on irritable bowel syndrome, fibromyalgia and chronic fatigue syndrome. *J Urology* 2010; *184*: 1358–1663.

Wallace DJ. Genitourinary manifestations of fibrositis: An increased association with the female urethral syndrome. *J Rheumatol 17*, 1990: 238–239.

Weiss JM. Chronic pelvic pain and myofascial trigger points. *The Pain Clinic* 2000; December, pp. 13–20.

14

Controversial Syndromes and Their Relationship to Fibromyalgia

It's no longer a question of staying healthy. It's a question of finding a sickness you like.

Jackie Mason (1931–)

Over the years, a variety of health professionals have developed terms or phrases to denote seemingly unique clinical combinations of symptoms and signs. A disorder or syndrome does not necessarily exist simply because it has been described in the medical literature. Some have stood the test of time, others overlap with syndromes described by different specialists, and additional terms may be favored by a single practitioner advocating a "cause." This chapter reviews conditions that have overlapping features with fibromyalgia but are not yet regarded as full-blown, legitimate disorders by organized medicine.

ALLERGIES AND "MULTIPLE CHEMICAL SENSITIVITY SYNDROME"

When Dr. Fine first met Wanda, she was a basket case. Wanda had canceled three prior appointments because smells from a new carpet had made her sick, medfly agricultural spraying 30 miles away prevented her from getting out of bed, and she developed a severe headache when her neighbors' house was being painted. She almost passed out in the elevator going to Dr. Fine's office because somebody was smoking. Wanda had been to three allergists, who obtained normal skin tests and blood tests. Desperate, she traveled to Mexico, where "immune rejuvenating" injections were administered, and to Texas, where a clinical ecologist sequestered her in a pollution-free, environmentally safe quonset hut for a month. There she received daily colonies, antiyeast medication, and vitamin shots, to no avail. Dr. Fine elicited a history of aching, sleep disorder, a "leaky gut," muscle pains, fatigue, and a spastic colon. His physical examination and mental status examination revealed evidence of anxiety, obsessive-compulsive tendencies, and fibromyalgia tender points. Wanda was treated with fluoxetine (Prozac) for pain and obsessive behavior, buspirone (Buspar), for anxiety during the day, and trazodone (Desyrel), a tricyclic, to help her sleep at night. She was referred to a psychologist who worked to improve Wanda's socialization skills and encouraged her to go out rather than be a prisoner in her own home. Wanda is slowly improving but will need many months of therapy.

Self-reported environmental sensitivities are observed in 15% of Americans. From 3% to 7% of fibromyalgia patients report extreme sensitivity to environmental components, particularly cigarette smoke, noise, bright lights, cold temperatures, pollution, gas, paint, perfumes, solvent fumes, pesticides, auto exhaust, certain foods, and carpet smells. A study conducted by the National Institutes of Health documented that one-half to three-quarters of patients with chronic fatigue syndrome (CFS) complain of having many allergies and sensitivities.

Multiple chemical sensitivity syndrome is a controversial entity. Proponents of the syndrome explain that it is triggered by exposure to diverse chemicals at doses lower than those documented to cause adverse affects in humans. They further define the condition as being reproducible with repeated chemical exposure of unrelated multiple substances that can affect multiple organs and symptoms that improve when the incitants are removed. Multiple chemical sensitivity is described as a acquired multi-organ condition where recurring symptoms include muscular weakness, confusion, memory loss, minor and major depression, general anxiety, panic, post-traumatic distress, respiratory distress, migratory joint pains, gastrointestinal and genitourinary malfunction, and "autoimmune" –like complaints. Inciting factors include common odorous substances (e.g., volatile organic compounds, perfumes, fresh paint, cleaning chemicals, print and toners, carpeting), drugs, water or food additives, and contaminants. *Cacosmia* is the subjective sense of feeling ill from low levels of environmental chemical odors. Interestingly, conventional allergy skin tests are usually normal.

Sensitivity related illnesses are defined as adverse clinical states elicited by exposure to low-dose diverse, environmental-borne physical chemical triggers and are self reported or objectively diagnosed responses. They have been termed *idiopathic environmental intolerances* by the World Health Organization and are also known as *medically unexplained syndromes.* Onset is related to different physical, chemical or biologic factors which include chemicals, drugs, metals, electro-magnetic or nuclear radiation, synthetic implants, specific foods, microbial, and environmental allergens.

About 5% of allergists call themselves *clinical ecologists* and attribute many of our nation's ills to environmental sensitivities. They use terms such as *chemically induced immune dysregulation, food allergies, leaky gut syndrome, allergic tension-fatigue syndrome, allergic toxemia, 20th-century disease, ecologic illness,* or *yeast syndrome* to explain these conditions. This group is not recognized by organized medicine and has developed testing methodologies that are not endorsed by mainstream practitioners. The National Research Council and the American Medical Association have issued position papers stating that there is not enough evidence to recognize multiple chemical sensitivity as a clinical syndrome. Many highly respected allergy/immunology specialists believe that multiple chemical sensitivity syndrome is overdiagnosed; others do not think it exists. This controversy is mentioned only to explain why some fibromyal gia patients may be given mixed signals and contradictory advice by various specialists.

Unfortunately, there is no consensus within the discipline of allergy and immunology about how to best define and categorize patients with environmental complaints who relate that allergies or chemicals cause widespread pain and fatigue. The American Academy of Allergy and Immunology, the American College of Physicians (to which most internists belong), and the American College of Occupational Medicine have issued position statements that the clinical ecology literature provides inadequate support for their beliefs and practices. In other words, evidence-based A level, double-blinded, prospective trials (in which patients did not know what they were being tested for or treated with and half of whom received no treatment) have not borne out clinical ecology theories.

Most patients labeled as having multiple chemical sensitivity syndrome have nociceptive amplification as a form of fibromyalgia or CFS, while others have a primary psychological disturbance, primarily a panic/anxiety disorder, which may play a role in these complaints. Additionally, we have had patients whose symptoms and signs disappeared with antiallergy therapies. Some "multiple chemical sensitivity" is not immunologic but a form of hypervigilance that results from the ability of the olfactory neurons and the limbic system to amplify responses to chemicals in concert with a dsyfunctioning ANS.

The most important issue in treating patients with environmental sensitivities and allergies is to make sure that they do not become so fearful of going outside and living normally that they become "environmental cripples."

A subset of patients with chemical sensitivity developed their condition, known as *sick building syndrome,* or *building-related illness,* after a defined exposure to microbes or allergens. Evaluating the structure's temperature, humidity, dust, formaldehyde, carbon monoxide, volatile and organic compounds is usually revealing. Because their fibromyalgia-like conditions evolved in numerous individuals after exposure to specific chemicals found in structures, this group of patients usually has a better prognosis than the overall multiple chemical sensitivity group in general.

Experimental data complicating the panic-anxiety mediated concept of multiple sensitivity syndrome is supportive of evidence that functional or genetic defects of enzymes detoxifying products of lipid peroxidation causes consequent metabolic and immunologic alterations via oxidative stress from environmental factors in some instances. No current "roadmap" exists to work up multiple chemical sensitivity complaints. Thus it may be difficult to sort out true environmental sensitivity from a psychiatric illness. A highly regarded group of immunologists in Israel led by Yehuda Shoenfeld has postulated that a condition termed *"ASIA"*, or *autoimmune/inflammatory syndrome* induced by adjuvants is responsible for Gulf War syndrome, siliconosis, macrophagic myofascitis syndrome, and post-vaccination phenomena among others (see below). Their theory has yet to be proven but may apply in certain circumstances.

Patients diagnosed with multiple chemical sensitivity syndrome should have their fibromyalgia managed symptomatically (see Parts VI and VII). They should work closely with their allergist/immunologist once a primary psychiatric disorder has been ruled out or treatment has been initiated (see Chapters 17 and 20).

GULF WAR SYNDROME

Approximately 70,000 of the 700,000 United States servicemen who served in the 1991 Persian Gulf War recorded complaints of fatigue (61%), nasal sinus congestion (51%), diarrhea (44%), joint stiffness, irritable colon, myalgias, cognitive impairment (41%), and headache (39%). When strict criteria were applied (symptoms starting two to three months after leaving the Persian Gulf with a duration of symptoms for six months, other diseases having been ruled out), approximately 20% fulfilled the ACR criteria for FM. An insect repellent known as DEET combined with pyridostigmine, an agent that minimizes the toxicity to nerve gas, was thought be a causative agent, but this was never confirmed.

A case definition which takes into account impaired cognition (distractibility, forgetfulness, depression, fatigue, daytime sleepiness, confusion-ataxia [reduced intellectual processing, confusion, vertigo, disorientation], and central pain [extremity joint pain, neck and shoulder pain, muscle and arm pain, numbness and tingling in the extremities] was found in 3.98% of nondeployed and 13.59% of deployed troops for an odds ratio of 3.87. Similar syndromes have been shown to occur following other wars.

SILICONOSIS

After graduating from high school, Tanya worked as a model. Although men found her quite attractive, her modeling roommates teased her about her small breasts. As Tanya was an only child from a broken home, these taunts did not help her self-image. On an impulse, she consulted a plastic surgeon who promised to make her a "complete woman." Tanya underwent breast augmentation with a silicone gel prosthesis. For five years the result looked great and she had few regrets, although she had some mild upper chest discomfort and the surgery had eliminated all nipple sensation. Then, over one–two years, symptoms of fatigue, burning, tingling, and aching started to evolve. Her eyes were so dry that she began using artificial tears. When press reports about silicone were published, Tanya went to a rheumatologist. Dr. Silbart obtained a positive antinuclear antibody (ANA) test and found evidence of fibromyalgia on physical examination. A plastic surgeon suspected a right-sided implant rupture that was confirmed on an MRI scan. After the implants were removed, Tanya's symptoms improved for about six months and her ANA level dropped by half. Her plastic surgeon and psychiatrist attributed her symptoms to Tanya's underlying psychological problems and felt strongly that the implant rupture was coincidental. Dr. Silbart believed that implants played an important role in her medical problems, but another rheumatologist referred by a law firm agreed with the psychiatrist and plastic surgeon. Her internist was not sure, and told Tanya that a combination of factors was causing her complaints, and reassured her in a way that minimized her anxieties and fears.

This controversial condition is based on the premise that the silicone in breast implants can be broken down to silica or related products, which spread throughout the body. For over 60 years, silica has been known to stimulate the immune system. Among exposed gold and uranium miners, silica occasionally results in the formation of autoantibodies and a scleroderma- or lupus-like disorder 10–30 years after exposure. *Siliconosis* could be its cousin seen in some patients with breast implants. Many siliconosis patients have a fibromyalgia-like condition with chronic fatigue, muscle and joint pain, swollen lymph glands, dry eyes, cognitive dysfunction, and difficulty swallowing, with or without the presence of autoantibodies. Other physicians have countered that silicone is not broken down to silica, and they believe that the role of these symptoms and illnesses is no different in women without implants. In the current litigious atmosphere, it will probably be several years before these claims are sorted out in a scientifically acceptable fashion, but the preponderance of evidence mitigates against siliconosis being a true entity.

LEAKY GUT SYNDROMES

Irritable bowel, spastic colitis, and functional bowel disease are recognized disorders of visceral hyperalgesia (increased pain sensitivity in internal structures), along with altered gut motility, and were reviewed in Chapter 13. Over the years, some homeopaths, naturopaths, and other alternative medicine practitioners have hypothesized that when too many substances pass through the lining of the small intestine, it becomes more permeable than usual. In other words, an overload of toxins or poisons is present that overwhelms the ability of the liver to detoxify them. As a consequence, inflammation and infections, as well as hormonal and neuromuscular changes, ensue.

Known as the *leaky gut syndrome,* this disorder has been held to cause *reactive hypoglycemia,* or low blood sugar, which in turn can induce palpitations, low blood pressure, and a feeling of faintness. Leaky gut syndrome has been claimed to be aggravated by aspirin- and ibuprofen-like products, food allergies, and yeast. Standard medical textbooks do not mention the existence of leaky gut syndrome, and most mainstream physicians believe that the majority of these patients have functional bowel or psychiatric disorders.

Candida Hypersensitivity Syndrome: A Yeast Connection or Disconnection?

Candida hypersensitivity syndrome is a variant of the leaky gut syndrome, according to Dr. William Crook, a Tennessee family practitioner, who popularized the theories of Dr. C. Orian Truss in a 1983 best-seller, *The Yeast Connection: A Medical Breakthrough.* Yeast is a fungus known by the technical term *candida.* The listing of functional bowel spectrum components in Table 13.4 of Chapter 13 should be considered in patients with "leaky gut" complaints.

Unfortunately, no controlled trials in the peer review literature support his claim, and when anti-yeast medication was given in a double-blind fashion (where half of the patients unknowingly took a placebo), no differences were noted. Yeast antibody tests are available in many clinical laboratories but consistently fail to identify patients who are infected—only those who have been exposed, which is virtually all of us. The American Academy of Allergy and Immunology issued a position paper stating that "the concept (of a yeast connection) is speculative and unproven..., elements of the proposed treatment program are potentially dangerous."

ARNOLD-CHIARI (CHIARI MALFORMATION) MYELOPATHY

Some of our patients have asked us if they qualify for the "surgical cure" of fibromyalgia. Such a cure does not exist, but desperate individuals sometimes undergo an expensive, painful procedure promoted by a few advocates that in our experience does not help the syndrome.

Syringomyelia and Chiari malformations are congenital or acquired disorders of the upper spine involving compression of nerves. Parts of the cerebellum (back of the brain) herniate into the spinal column and compress the brainstem, which produces headaches, burning and shooting pains in the back and neck, fatigue, vertigo, hearing loss, blurred or double vision, and a staggering gait. As usually performed, CT or MR imaging of the neck and brain rarely show this condition unless special views are ordered. These seriously ill patients do not have fibromyalgia, but a compressive myelopathy that mimics it. They benefit from decompressive surgery, but the condition is relatively rare.

Some individuals with Chiari malformations have been *misdiagnosed* as having fibromyalgia. If your family doctor finds very brisk reflexes or a Babinski reflex on a routine examination and the above complaints are present, a Chiari work-up is indicated. Nearly all patients with Chiari malformations have this easy-to-find neurologic testing abnormality. Studies of fibromyalgia patients found no differences in abnormalities in brain and spine imaging consistent with Chiari malformations compared with a control group. Many healthy people (and patients with fibromyalgia) have slight imaging abnormalities suggesting an asymptomatic, mild Chiari-like compression.

MERCURY AMALGAMS

The use of mercury-silver amalgam fillings in the mouth has been held to produce chronic fatigue, headaches, cognitive dysfunction, and muscle and joint aches. Although the American Dental Association considers mercury amalgams to be a safe, effective method of tooth restoration, there may be an extremely small group of patients who are sensitive to this product. A large scale study showed no evidence that mercury amalgams are toxic.

SUMMING UP

If you have been diagnosed as having multiple chemical sensitivity syndrome, Gulf War syndrome, siliconosis, a leaky gut with or without yeast infection, mercury amalgam toxicity, Chiari malformation, or interstitial cystitis, be aware that these diagnoses are controversial and may not truly exist. Before initiating expensive, time-consuming, toxic, or lifestyle-altering therapies that are unproven, make sure that your treating physicians agree on the best course of action to take. Or at least, look before you leap!

FOR FURTHER READING

AMA Council of Scientific Affairs. Clinical ecology. *JAMA 268*, 1992: 3465–3467.

Bellinger DC, Trachtenberg F, Barregard L, *et al.* Neuropsychological and renal effects of dental amalgam in children: A randomized controlled trial, *JAMA* 2006; *295*: 1775–1783.

De Luca C, Raskovic D, Pacifico V, *et al.* The search for reliable biomarkers of disease in multiple chemical sensitivity and other environmental intolerances. *Int J Environ Res Public Health* 2011; *8*: 2770–2797.

Iannacchione VG, Dever JA, Bann CM, *et al.* Validation of research case definition of Gulf War illness in the 1991 US military population. *Neuroepidemiology* 2011; *37*: 129–140.

Menzies D, Bourbeau J. Building-related illnesses. *N Engl J Med* 1997; *338*: 1524–1531.

Shoenfeld Y, Agmon-Levin N. "ASIA"—autoimmune/inflammatory syndrome induced by adjuvants. *J Autoimmun* 2011; *36*: 4–8.

Watson NF, Buchwald D, Goldberg J, *et al.* Is Chiari I malformation associated with fibromyalgia? *Neurosurgery* 2011; *68*: 443–448.

Part V
THE EVALUATION
OF FIBROMYALGIA
PATIENTS

Patients with fibromyalgia-related symptoms may consult a variety of health care professionals and physicians in all specialties. This part reviews what patients and doctors look for, what tests are ordered, and how they are interpreted. How can a doctor be sure that the diagnosis is correct? Is another diagnosis being missed? And finally, is it really all in one's head?

15

What Happens at a Fibromyalgia Consultation?

We don't believe in rheumatism and true love until after the first attack.
Marie von Ebner-Eschenbach (1830–1916)

Fibromyalgia is usually a diagnosis of exclusion. Often poorly understood by some primary care physicians, the diagnosis of fibromyalgia is often delayed. Even though in one survey up to 10% of general medical visits involve a complaint of generalized musculoskeletal pain, the diagnosis was made only after patients saw a mean of 3.5 doctors. This chapter will take you through the workup that establishes the definitive diagnosis and eliminates other possible explanations for the patient's complaints.

WHO SHOULD BE THE FIBROMYALGIA CONSULTANT AND HOW CAN THE PATIENT PREPARE FOR THE VISIT?

Doctors who diagnose and treat fibromyalgia often cross specialty lines. Although rheumatologists tend to regard fibromyalgia as residing within their bailiwick, there are too few of us to handle all the needs of the six million fibromyalgia sufferers. The 5,000 rheumatologists in clinical practice in the United States are internal medicine subspecialists. A total of 200,000 doctors practice primary care internal medicine or family practice in the United States, and are front line doctors for most patients. These physicians may suspect fibromyalgia and consult a rheumatologist to confirm the diagnosis. In complicated cases, the rheumatologist can take over the management of the condition. Orthopedists, neurosurgeons, and neurologists frequently diagnose fibromyalgia but generally refer patients to rheumatologists or internists for treatment. Rheumatologists may refer patients to physical medicine specialists or pain management centers when their approaches do not bear fruit.

Suppose that you are suspected of having fibromyalgia, and a primary care physician has referred you to a fibromyalgia consultant (usually a rheumatologist but sometimes an internist, physiatrist, neurologist, orthopedist, or osteopath) to confirm the diagnosis and make management suggestions. Is any

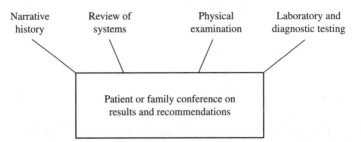

Fig. 15.1. *The fibromyalgia consultation. (From D. J. Wallace, The Lupus Book. New York: Oxford University Press, 1995, p. 123; reprinted with permission.)*

sort of advanced preparation advisable? Yes. Bring copies of outside records and previous test results or work-ups to the consultant. If you have more than a few complaints or are taking more than a few medications, a summary list is useful. The evaluation will consist of a history, physical examination, diagnostic laboratory tests, and possibly imaging studies (X-rays, scans, etc.). Once all the observations and test results are in, the doctor will discuss the findings with you—perhaps at the time of the visit, by telephone after the initial meeting, or in a follow-up visit. The consultation process is illustrated in Figure 15.1.

DR. WALLACE'S CONSULTATION: PATIENT INTERVIEW

I begin by asking why the patient has come in and how he or she feels. Once I've heard the patient's symptoms and history, I conduct a review of systems. As many as 100 questions can be asked as part of the screening process. Positive responses may lead to an additional set of queries that clarify symptoms in a given area, such as how long the complaint has been present, whether it is constant or intermittent, what time of day it is present, what makes it better or worse, how it has been diagnostically evaluated and treated in the past, and the current status.

I ask the patient about allergies and about family members' history of rheumatic disease or other diseases. Other relevant facts include possible occupational exposure to allergic or toxic substances, a detailed description of what his or her body does during the day, how much and what exercise or activities are performed, educational attainment, and with whom the patient lives. Unusual childhood diseases are also explored, as well as tobacco or alcohol use and abuse, immunizations, previous hospitalization and surgeries, past and present prescriptions, and frequency of use of over-the-counter medications. These questions also provide the basis of a psychosocial profile, which may be important in developing a productive doctor-patient relationship.

The internal medicine/rheumatic review of systems covers these categories:

1. *Constitutional symptoms,* such as fevers, malaise, weight loss, or swollen glands, are dealt with first. They refer to the patient's overall state and how he or she feels. This is followed by an organ system review that goes from head to toe.
2. The *head and neck* review includes inquiries about cataracts, glaucoma, dry eyes, dry mouth, eye pain, jaw pain, double vision, loss of vision, iritis, conjunctivitis, ringing in the ears, loss of hearing, frequent ear infections, frequent nosebleeds, smell abnormalities, frequent sinus infections, sores in the nose or mouth, dental problems, or swollen glands in the neck.
3. The *cardiopulmonary* system is covered next. I ask about asthma, bronchitis, emphysema, tuberculosis, pleurisy (pain on taking a deep breath), shortness of breath, pneumonia, high blood pressure, chest pains, rheumatic fever, heart murmur, heart attack, palpitations, and irregular heartbeat.
4. The *gastrointestinal* system review includes an effort to find any evidence of swallowing difficulties, severe nausea or vomiting, diarrhea, constipation, unusual eating habits, hepatitis, bloating, flatulence, ulcers, gallstones, blood in stool or vomit, diverticulitis, colitis, or pancreatitis.
5. The *genitourinary* area should be approached in a respectful, sensitive way. In addition to inquiring about frequent bladder infections, kidney stones, prostate problems, or blood or protein in the urine, I review the obstetrical history, breast disorders, and menstrual problems.
6. Next, the *hematologic* and *immune* factors that the patient may be aware of include how easily he or she bruises, anemia, low white blood cell or platelet counts, and frequent infections.
7. A *neuropsychiatric* history takes into account headaches, seizures, numbness or tingling, fainting, psychiatric or antidepressant interventions, substance abuse, difficulty sleeping, and cognitive dysfunction. If it is relevant and I feel comfortable approaching the subject, sexual dysfunction, a history of sexual abuse, domestic violence, or physical abuse may be reviewed. This may also be the time to inquire about blood transfusions or even AIDS risk factors.
8. *Musculoskeletal* concerns involve a history of joint pain, stiffness, gout, muscle pains, or weakness and better characterization of the complaints of fibromyalgia.
9. The *endocrine* system review includes questions about thyroid disease, diabetes, and high cholesterol level.
10. The *vascular* history may uncover prior episodes of phlebitis, clots, swelling, fluid retention, strokes, or Raynaud's phenomenon (fingers turning different colors in cold weather).

11. Finally, the *skin* is discussed. Evidence of sun sensitivity, hair loss, mouth sores, rashes. Psoriasis, eczema, or changes in skin coloring are carefully reviewed.

In concluding the history taking, I always ask the patient whether there is anything I should know that was not covered. One of my mentors, Edmund Dubois, devoted his rheumatology textbook to "the patients, from whom we have learned." Physicians become better doctors when they listen to what patients have to say about things that the doctor may not have brought up. Occasionally, the patient mentions something in a casual conversation that turns out to be quite important in shedding light on his or her health problems.

THE PHYSICAL EXAMINATION

The history and review of systems elucidate what physicians call *symptoms;* physical examination reveals *signs.* Four methods known as *inspection* (looking at an area), *palpation* (feeling an area), *percussion* (gentle knocking against a surface such as the lung or liver to detect fullness or size), and *auscultation* (listening with a stethoscope to the heart, chest, carotid artery, etc.) are employed during the complete physical. Patients are evaluated from head to toe.

First, *vital signs* are checked to ascertain weight, pulse, respirations, blood pressure, and temperature. The *head and neck* exam includes evaluation of the pupils' response to light, eye movements, cataracts, and vessels of the eye. The ear exam searches for obstruction and inflammation. The oral cavity is screened for sores, poor dental hygiene, and dryness. I palpate the thyroid and the glands of the neck and also listen to the neck for abnormal murmurs or sounds (carotid artery bruits). The *chest* examination consists of inspection (e.g., for postural abnormalities), palpation for chest wall tenderness, percussion to detect fluid in the lungs, and auscultation (e.g., to rule out asthma or pneumonia). The *heart* is checked for murmurs, clicks, or irregular beats. The *abdomen* is inspected for obesity, distention, or scars; palpated for pain or hernia; percussed to assess the size of the liver and spleen; and auscultated to rule out any obstruction or vascular sounds. This is followed by an *extremity* evaluation, which includes looking for swelling, color changes, inflamed joints, and deformities. Specific maneuvers allow me to assess range of motion, muscle strength, pulses, muscle tone, and fibromyalgia tender points. If indicated, a genitourinary evaluation is done. It includes a breast examination, rectal evaluation, and pelvic examination (in women a Pap smear and in men a prostate exam). In rheumatology, a genitourinary exam is necessary only if the patient has complaints relevant to these areas and no other physician has recently performed one. A *neurobehavioral* assessment reflecting change in mental status is usually conducted as part of the ongoing conversation; neurologic deficits can be detected by observing the patient for tremor, gait abnormalities, or abnormal sensation, movements, or reflexes. Finally, the *skin* is examined for rashes, pigment changes, tattoos, hair loss, Raynaud's phenomenon, and skin breakdown or ulcerations.

The physical examination may include other steps as well, depending upon the problem reported and the nature of the consultation. A thorough physical examination is usually conducted after a detailed interview and allows me to order appropriate tests.

MUST BLOOD BE DRAWN OR URINE EXAMINED?

A history and physical examination may suggest the diagnosis of fibromyalgia, but in order to make sure that other disorders with complaints and physical findings similar to those of fibromyalgia are not present, it is necessary to perform blood laboratory tests.

When a patient arrives at an internist's or family practitioner's office for a general medical evaluation, it usually includes what doctors refer to as *screening laboratory tests*. In other words, by obtaining a blood count, urine test, and blood chemistry panel, abnormalities can be detected in 90% of individuals with serious medical problems. All the tests listed below are inexpensive and mostly automated; they can be performed within hours and do not require special expertise. Most large medical offices are equipped to perform these tests on the premises. In fibromyalgia the tests are almost always normal.

A *complete blood count* (CBC) analyzes your red blood cells, white blood cells, and platelets (which are responsible for clotting). The CBC screens for anemia, infections, risk factors for infection, and bleeding disorders. *Blood chemistry* panels consist of anywhere from 7 to 25 tests that evaluate a variety of parameters, including blood sugar, kidney function (blood urea nitrogen [BUN], creatinine), liver function (aspartate aminotransferase [AST], alanine aminotransferase [ALT], bilirubin, alkaline phosphatase, gamma glutamyl-transferase [GGT]), electrolytes (sodium, potassium, chloride, bicarbonate, calcium, phosphorus, magnesium), lipids or fats (cholesterol, triglycerides, high density lipoprotein [HDL], low density lipoprotein [LDL]), proteins (albumin, total protein), thyroid function (triiodothyronine [T_3], thyroxine [T_4], thyroid-stimulating hormone [TSH]), and gout (uric acid). Occasionally chemistry panels include additional studies (amylase for pancreatic function, lactic dehydrogenase [LDH] for red blood cell breakdown, iron or vitamin B_{12} levels), which are also inexpensive and can be added upon request. Other inexpensive blood tests that may be asked for include a creatine phosphokinase (CPK) to rule out muscle inflammation, a Westergren sedimentation rate or C-reactive protein test to rule out inflammation in the bloodstream or tissues, and tests for clotting time (prothrombin time [PT], partial thromboplastin time [PTT], bleeding time). A *urinalysis* is a useful screen for kidney disease, kidney stones, urinary tract infections, and other conditions.

WHEN ARE IMAGING STUDIES, ELECTRICAL EVALUATIONS, AND SPECIALIZED BLOOD TESTS REQUESTED?

When evaluating a potential fibromyalgia patient, I usually obtain a chest X-ray and EGG of the heart if one has not been done recently. These are also inexpensive and safe procedures that rule out potentially important causes of chest area pains, palpitations, and shortness of breath.

In certain circumstances, additional blood testing may be useful. Autoimmune blood tests consisting of an ANA or rheumatoid factor screen for systemic lupus and rheumatoid arthritis may be necessary. If these tests are positive, as they are in a small number of fibromyalgia patients, specific additional ANA panels can be obtained to confirm the diagnosis. Fibromyalgia patients frequently complain of numbness, tingling, and burning. The doctor may want to get X-rays (and, if abnormal, an MRI or computed tomography [CT] scan) of the neck or low back to make sure that a bone spur or herniated disc is not causing these symptoms. An EMG can also diagnose herniated discs or indicate if numbness is from carpal tunnel syndrome, diabetes, or an inflammatory process. Bone scans can look for tumors or inflammation. Sleep EEGs (polysomnography) may be ordered if it is important to document a physiologic basis for complaints of unrefreshing sleep.

There are additional blood tests, imaging, and electrical studies that are inexpensive and useful and may be appropriate in specific situations. Some of them are reviewed in the next chapter.

ARE THERE UNPROVEN DIAGNOSTIC TESTS?

Occasionally, doctors order tests that are not necessary and others that have no known value. Unproven testing consists of procedures that needlessly run up the bill, are never helpful in the diagnosis and/or treatment of the patient, are not covered by insurance companies, and are considered invalid by most doctors. Few of these studies will change anything a knowledgeable doctor would do for the patient. In patients with probable primary fibromyalgia, I see no reason to order T- and B-cell counts with lymphocyte subsets; tests for mitogenic stimulation; yeast antibody levels; nail, hair, or body chemical analysis; cytotoxic testing; skin endpoint titration; provocation-neutralization testing; or a food immune complex assay. Check out a doctor's credentials before taking the plunge. Call your local hospital, medical association, or university. Is the doctor board-certified by a specialty recognized by the American College of Physicians or the American Board of Medical Specialties?

SUMMING UP

If a primary care doctor has referred a patient to a qualified specialist to confirm a diagnosis or make suggestions on how to manage fibromyalgia, it's helpful for the patient to be organized, direct, and have easy-to-digest summaries of past and present medical complaints, prior blood tests, imaging or electrical evaluations, and treatments. The specialist will perform a comprehensive evaluation, which should provide the primary care doctor with the consultation or information needed to assure patients of the highest quality care.

16

Are You Sure It's Really Fibromyalgia?

Ever since I have been ill, I have longed and longed for some palpable disease, no matter how conventionally dreadful a label it might have, but I was always driven back to stagger alone under the monstrous mass of subjective sensations, which that sympathetic being, "The Medicine Man," had no higher inspiration than to assure me I was personally responsible for, washing his hands of me with a graceful complacency.

Alice James (1848–1892), *The Diary of Alice James*

A week doesn't go by without a patient wanting my reassurance that he or she is not seriously ill or making it all up. "Are you just telling me it's fibromyalgia because you don't want me to be upset?" "A friend of mine told me that fibromyalgia is a 'garbage can' diagnosis that doctors give when they don't know what you have." These are frequent remarks or queries. How is your doctor really sure that something is not being missed? This chapter reviews some diseases with features that can overlap with or be mistaken for fibromyalgia.

FIBROMYALGIA CAN BE PART OF OTHER DISEASES

Fibromyalgia can seem to be working in concert with other diseases. For example, untreated inflammation associated with an autoimmune disease (such as rheumatoid arthritis or systemic lupus erythematosus), other forms of inflammatory arthritis (such as ankylosing spondylitis), or a chest disease known as *sarcoidosis* are associated with coexisting fibromyalgia. Withdrawal from or tapering of medications such as corticosteroids typically precipitates or aggravates fibromyalgia. Approximately 13% of FM patients were originally diagnosed as having another rheumatic disease and vice versa.

SOME DISORDERS CAN MIMIC OR INTERACT WITH FIBROMYALGIA

Many disorders interact with or can be mistaken for fibromyalgia. They are reviewed here, as well as in other parts of this book, and listed in Table 16.1.

Table 16.1. *Common Disorders that Can Mimic Fibromyalgia*

Hormonal imbalances
  Menstrual disorders
  Low thyroid, high parathyroid levels
  Pregnancy
  Adrenal insufficiency
  Diabetes
  Menopause
  Low Vitamin D
Infections
  Bacteria
  Viruses
  Fungi
  Parasites
Musculoskeletal or autoimmune disorders
  Rheumatoid arthritis
  Ankylosing spondylitis in females
  Seronegative spondyloarthropathies
  Lyme disease
  Systemic lupus erythematosus
  Palindromic rheumatism
  Inflammatory bowel disease
  Polymyalgia rheumatica
  Celiac disease
  Sjogren's syndrome
  Generalized osteoarthritis
Neurologic disease
  Peripheral neuropathy
  Multiple sclerosis
  Myasthenia gravis
Malignancy
Substance abuse
Malnutrition
Primary psychiatric disorders
Allergies
Anemia

Hormonal Imbalances

Linda was not herself. Over a period of several months, she found it increasingly difficult to make it through the day. Her muscles started to ache, she gained 15 pounds while on the same diet, found it difficult to tolerate cold weather, and her voice became husky. Dr. Bridges did a complete blood count and a blood panel that was normal. He was impressed with her muscle aches and diagnosed her as having fibromyalgia. When Dr. White saw Linda in a rheumatology consultation, certain things did not fit. Weight gain, a hoarse voice, and cold intolerance of recent onset are not typical features of fibromyalgia, so she obtained additional tests that included a complete thyroid panel (triiodothyronine [T_3], thyroxine [T_4], thyroid-stimulating hormone [TSH]). Although the T_3 and T_4 levels were normal (as they had been with Dr. Bridges), the TSH (which was not part of Dr. Bridges's panel) was quite high, indicating hypothyroidism. Linda was started on thyroid replacement therapy and was back to herself within a few weeks.

Low *thyroid* levels, or *hypothyroidism* can be mistaken for fibromyalgia. Blood T_3, T_4, and TSH tests readily and inexpensively differentiate these disorders. *Parathyroid tumors* or adenomas raise blood calcium levels and cause aching, weakness, and palpitations. The parathyroid gland overlies the thyroid, and disorders of this gland are detected by measuring calcium, phosphorus, and parathormone blood levels. *Adrenal glands* overlie the kidney and make cortisone. Adrenal insufficiency (Addison's disease) or adrenal overactivity (Cushing's disease) can modulate fibromyalgia symptoms. *Diabetics* with peripheral nerve disease complain of numbness and tingling. If their sugar level is too high or too low, they complain of fatigue, palpitations, and weakness. Low *vitamin D* levels are associated with musculoskeletal pain.

Hormonal disorders produce fatigue, aching, and weakness. *Premenstrual syndrome (PMS)* frequently aggravates fibromyalgia symptoms. *Menopause* can improve fibromyalgia, but early menopausal symptoms can mimic and aggravate the syndrome. Irregular periods, use of birth control pills, and painful periods may produce symptoms of bloating, fatigue, and aching. It is also important to make sure that new fibromyalgia-like symptoms are not in fact an early *pregnancy.*

Infections

Bacteria, viruses, fungi, parasites, and other microbes infect the body and produce a variety of systemic reactions, including fatigue, malaise, fevers, swollen glands, rashes, joint pain, shortness of breath, abdominal pain, and difficulty thinking clearly. Infections and fibromyalgia can interact in three different ways: postinfectious fatigue syndromes can cause fibromyalgia and chronic fatigue syndrome, fibromyalgia may be mistaken for infection and vice versa, and infections can aggravate fibromyalgia.

A doctor can screen for infections with the work-up reviewed in the previous chapter but may need additional tests. These may include cultures of blood, urine, sputum, stool, bone marrow, skin lesions, spinal fluid, pleural fluid, or whatever bodily tissues are accessible, and serum antibody levels to organisms to ascertain prior or current exposure. Sometimes, doctors perform skin tests (such as a tuberculosis skin test) or order scans to identify infected areas. Infections should be promptly identified and treated.

Musculoskeletal Disorders

As mentioned earlier, 7–22% of patients with autoimmune diseases have secondary fibromyalgia and may be mistakenly diagnosed as having the syndrome.

Early *rheumatoid arthritis* sometimes appears fibromyalgia-like before it settles in the hands and feet and causes joint swelling. *Systemic lupus erythematosus* is commonly misdiagnosed as fibromyalgia because overlapping fatigue, aching, and cognitive impairment symptoms can be confusing. Ten million Americans have a positive ANA, which is almost always seen in lupus, but only one million Americans have lupus. Therefore, patients who present to a rheumatologist with a positive ANA and nonspecific symptoms often go through a work-up to rule out lupus, which may include obtaining muscle enzymes, inflammatory indices such as sedimentation rate, skin biopsy specimens, bone scans, and detailed autoantibody blood testing. *Polymyositis* is an inflammatory muscle disease differentiated from fibromyalgia by elevation of the muscle enzyme *creatine phosphokinase* in blood testing.

Rheumatoid variants such as *ankylosing spondylitis, psoriatic arthritis, arthritis of inflammatory bowel disease, undifferentiated spondyloarthropathies* and *reactive arthritis* may be hard to distinguish from fibromyalgia since they are often only intermittently inflammatory. Many rheumatoid variant patients have a positive blood test for a marker known as HLA-B27. *Palindromic rheumatism* presents as a pre-rheumatoid arthritis, prelupus-like condition, with infrequent physical findings of joint swelling and symptoms of aching and fatigue. *Polymyalgia rheumatica* is seen in older patients who have aching in their shoulder and hip areas; it is usually easy to differentiate from fibromyalgia since the blood sedimentation rate is elevated. FM rarely responds to anti-inflammatory therapies.

Hypermobility syndromes and *work overuse syndromes* may be misdiagnosed as fibromyalgia but are associated with regional myofascial syndromes, as are *osteoarthritis, spinal stenosis,* and *disc problems* in the cervical and lumbar spines. Most people in their 40s and 50s have nonspecific abnormalities on X-rays or CT or MRI scans, and sometimes low back pain or neck pain is interpreted as a herniated disc when it is really due to fibromyalgia. Low back pain costs Americans $100 billion a year. Eighty percent of this amount is incurred by 5% of those with low back pain, in some of whom the diagnosis of fibromyalgia is overlooked.

NEUROLOGIC DISEASE

Tina was a tireless housewife who always did three things at once. One day, she dropped the bag she was carrying from the car while experiencing a "weak spell." Over the following weeks, Tina noticed some numbness and tingling in her legs that her husband thought could be a herniated disc from her vigorous workout. Her family doctor was not sure what the problem was and made an offhand remark that it could be due to a flu or a type of fibromyalgia. Over the next week, Tina became unsteady as she walked and complained of being dizzy. An MRI scan of her brain was diagnostic for multiple sclerosis, and she was referred to a neurologist for treatment.

Patients with early forms of *multiple sclerosis* and *myasthenia gravis* complain of numbness, aching, fatigue, weakness, and difficulty thinking clearly without dramatic physical findings. Unlike fibromyalgia, multiple sclerosis is characterized by MRI and spinal fluid abnormalities, and myasthenia gravis is marked by abnormal electrical studies and positive antibody tests. To further confuse the issue, secondary fibromyalgia accompanies neurologic disease in up to 20% of these patients. Primary muscle or nerve disorders associated with complaints of numbness, tingling, or burning can be differentiated from fibromyalgia by EMG and nerve conduction studies, as well as by various forms of spinal imaging. Nerve or muscle biopsies are occasionally recommended to clarify the diagnosis.

Malignancies

Patients with cancer make a variety of extra chemicals, many of which cause systemic symptoms, including fatigue, aching, and weakness, that resemble fibromyalgia complaints. These *paraneoplastic* features of a tumor usually disappear with treatment including chemotherapy, radiation therapy, and surgery. Steroids frequently are used along with chemotherapy, and disease onset and/or changes can produce fibromyalgia. Selected drugs used to treat cancer, such as *alpha-interferon* (for hepatitis or leukemia) or *interleukin-2* (e.g., for melanoma or kidney cancer) may induce fibromyalgia-like symptoms that last for weeks to months. Healthy-appearing young women with early stages of *Hodgkin's disease* and other *lymphomas* initially have been diagnosed incorrectly as having fibromyalgia.

Substance Abuse and Malnutrition

Things were not going well for Kelly. Although her fibromyalgia was under fair control, Kelly always seemed tired. She never appeared to eat regularly, and her weight dropped below 100 pounds. Kelly was becoming an alcoholic. When the judge cut her divorce payments by half and her children left for college, Kelly advanced from being a social drinker at night to consuming cocktails whenever she could. It took a while for her friends to catch on. Kelly was very good at hiding her habit and drank six to eight cups of coffee or cola drinks a day. She stole diet pills from her friends' medicine cabinets to give her more energy. Kelly's self-destructive actions persisted until her three best friends took her to Spa Ranch near Death Valley, California, for a weekend. Kelly promptly convulsed from alcohol withdrawal and was cut off from her caffeine and stimulants. At the nearby community hospital, Kelly's fibromyalgia pain was excruciating. After she returned home, her family physician helped her enter the Alcoholics Anonymous program, and she graduated successfully from the 12-step program. Her muscles now rarely hurt, and she is receiving counseling.

Our society provides many means—legal and otherwise—to obtain agents that can produce or alleviate fatigue. Caffeine is an addictive chemical in coffee, tea, headache formulas (e.g., Excedrin, Fioricet), and cola beverages that can increase the heart rate. People who are dependent on caffeine develop fatigue and palpitations or withdrawal symptoms when they are deprived of it for a day or two. Many of these individuals take diet pills or "uppers" to manage fatigue, which can also lead to appetite loss, weight loss, and malnutrition.

The number of patients who complain of profound fatigue and do not realize (or deny) that it could be due to taking high doses of prescription painkillers such as Vicodin, codeine, Darvon, or Percocet is amazing. Alcohol, cocaine, and heroin abuse are common causes of fatigue, but dependence on pain medicine is very common. Sudden withdrawal of any of these substances is associated with pain amplification. Finally, the presence of significant, unintentional weight loss, fever, swollen joints, rashes, enlarged lymph glands, or focal neurologic signs should alert patients and physicians that an alternative or additional diagnosis is probable.

DEAR DOCTOR: THINK OF FIBROMYALGIA

Make no mistake about it. Fibromyalgia will never be diagnosed unless a doctor considers it to be a diagnostic possibility. Many doctors were trained before accepted definitions and criteria for the syndrome were established. We have seen many patients who had cancer and infection work-ups, expensive MRI and CT scans, adrenal evaluations, and even surgical procedures when a better-focused work-up would have revealed the real problem. Managed care has caused many doctors to think twice before ordering these expensive studies or asking for help from a consultant. "Megawork-ups" will decrease over the next few years as our health care environment changes and continuing medical education for physicians becomes more widespread.

SUMMING UP

Fibromyalgia is a diagnosis of exclusion. Serious and treatable disorders with overlapping symptoms and signs should be ruled out before patients are convinced and the doctor feels comfortable with the diagnosis. If a patient has fibromyalgia secondary to one of several disorders, it won't get better until the primary or underlying disease is addressed. Doctors try their best, but the patient's symptoms, signs, and physical findings can be subtle and don't always lead directly to a diagnosis of fibromyalgia.

FOR FURTHER READING

Di Franco M, Iannuccelli C, Bazzichi L, *et al.* Misdiagnosis of fibromyalgia: a multicenter study, *Clin Exp Rheumatol* 2011; *29* (S69): S104–S108.

Eraso RM, Bradford NJ, Fontenot CN, *et al.* Fibromyalgia in young children: onset at age 10 years and younger, *Clin Exp Rheumatol* 2007; *25*: 639–644.

Hench PK. Evaluation and differential diagnosis of fibromyalgia. *Med Clin NA 15*, 1989: 19–30.

17
I'm Not Crazy!

A bodily disease, which we look upon as whole and entire within itself may,
after all, be but a symptom of some ailment in the spiritual part.

Nathaniel Hawthorne (1804–1864)

"You look fine, and I can't find anything wrong with you. Maybe you're just depressed or stressed out." Nearly all of my patients have heard this before. And they start to wonder: Am I really crazy? How could it all be in my mind? This chapter will summarize the small number of behavioral surveys that rheumatologists and psychiatrists have performed on fibromyalgia patients. The treatment of fibromyalgia will be reviewed in Parts VI and VII.

Why are there so few studies that we can rely upon? First, most research is conducted at university medical centers, where fibromyalgia patients tend to be more symptomatic and have not responded to interventions by community physicians. Second, depression itself is associated with high rates of musculoskeletal pain. Also, few people have had comprehensive psychological evaluations *before* they became ill that can be used for comparison. Finally, instruments of psychological assessment were devised before we knew what fibromyalgia was, and popular tests such as the Minnesota Multiphasic Personality Inventory (MMPI) cannot distinguish between pain from a disease and pain from depression.

DO I HURT BECAUSE I'M DEPRESSED OR AM I DEPRESSED BECAUSE I HURT?

Is fibromyalgia a manifestation of depression or the reverse? Well-designed studies have addressed this issue, but many used different methods, populations, ethnic groupings, referral sources, and geographical distributions. In any case, the results were reasonably similar. On average, these studies showed that about 18% of fibromyalgia patients have evidence of a major depression at any office visit and 58% have a history of major depression in their lifetime. What does this mean? *At any point in time, the overwhelming majority of fibromyalgia patients are not seriously depressed.* And if they are depressed, it's usually because they do not feel well. This condition is called *reactive depression* and is reversible with treatment, as opposed to *endogenous depression*, which is caused by chemical imbalances and is much harder to treat. A well-designed study of depressed patients demonstrated that fewer than 10% had two or more tender points.

ARE THERE HISTORICAL BEHAVIORAL FACTORS THAT ARE MORE COMMON IN FIBROMYALGIA PATIENTS THAN IN THOSE WITHOUT THE DISORDER?

Certain life events or historical factors are statistically present more often in fibromyalgia patients than in those without the disorder. This does not mean that more than a minority of patients have had these problems. Statistical methods have allowed us to do *case control studies,* in which each fibromyalgia patient is matched with a person without fibromyalgia who is of the same age, race, and sex. Some case control studies also match geographic locations, educational backgrounds, socioeconomic status, and other factors. One popular method is for each patient in a study to pick a healthy friend as the control. Mathematical formulas allow surveyors to devise a *relative risk* or *odds ratio.* For example, a survey might determine in a case-controlled fashion that a patient is twice as likely to have a family history of alcoholism or cancer as a friend with a relative risk of 2.0, or 2 to 1. This, for example, makes the odds twice as likely that fibromyalgia patients will have these features.

Studies conducted in the last few years show that fibromyalgia patients have a significantly increased risk of having a history of sexual, physical, or drug abuse, eating disorders, mood disorders, attention deficit disorder, phobias (unrealistic fears), panic, anxiety, somatization, and a family history of depression or alcoholism. They also show that fibromyalgia patients cope less well with daily problems than others and are more susceptible to psychological stress. We have already shown that psychological stress can lower the pain threshold. Certain studies also suggest that there is more *alexithymia,* a longstanding personality disorder with generalized and localized complaints in individuals who cannot express their underlying psychological conflicts. As a consequence, some behavioral experts have proposed that fibromyalgia is an *affective spectrum disorder* in which a primary psychiatric disorder with a possibly inherited abnormality leads to pain amplification and fibromyalgia-related complaints.

WHAT'S WRONG WITH THE AFFECTIVE SPECTRUM MODEL OF FIBROMYALGIA?

These studies promoted an intense debate among fibromyalgia experts as to whether fibromyalgia is a manifestation of a *psychological* disturbance or a *physiological* disorder of pain amplification. We strongly believe that the latter explanation is more accurate. Why do we feel so strongly? First, biochemical abnormalities (e.g., increased substance P level in spinal fluid, abnormal functional brain imaging, genetic polymorphisms that increase sensitivity to pain) have been found in fibromyalgia that do not correlate with behavioral abnormalities (Figure 17.1). Second, fibromyalgia frequently occurs in conditions such as scoliosis, which have never been associated with any behavioral disorders. Third, all of the behavioral surveys supporting an affective spectrum disorder were performed at university medical centers and do not reflect what an internist or family physician sees in a community fibromyalgia population practice. For example, sexual abuse may be one of *many* triggers or aggravating factors of fibromyalgia syndrome, but it is seen in a small number of patients with the syndrome. For most patients followed in a community practice, the syndrome is not serious enough for them to be referred to a specialist. Specialists generally deal with more severe cases, which skews their study results. A landmark study by Dr. Larry Bradley at the University of Alabama has clearly proven this point. *Though more patients with fibromyalgia have a history of psychosocial distress than patients with some other musculoskeletal conditions, this does not explain*

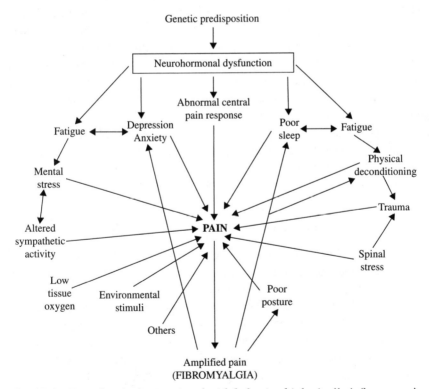

Fig. 17.1. *How chemicals associated with behavior biologically influence pain.*

why a majority of individuals with fibromyalgia have no significant psychoso-cial distress.

FIBROMYALGIA PERSONALITY PROFILES

In the morning she was asked how she slept. "Oh terribly badly!" said the Princess. "I have scarcely shut my eyes the whole night. Heaven only knows what was in the bed, but I was lying on something hard, so that I am black and blue all over." Nobody but a real princess could be as sensitive as that. So the prince took her for his wife, for now he knew he had a real princess.

Hans Christian Andersen (1805–1875),
The Princess and the Pea, 1835

In our opinion, patients with fibromyalgia tend to have several personality pro-files. At least half with the syndrome are females, aged 20–60, who have above average intelligence. They display perfectionistic tendencies, are efficient, well groomed, like to be organized, in control, and often make lists. An inciting event such as infection, trauma, new work responsibilities, or family pressures or stresses upset a delicate balance. Because they fear failure, rejection, or feel guilty because it's increasingly difficult to maintain their current lifestyle and activities, a preexisting mild, chronic anxiety gets worse. This makes it difficult to sleep and ultimately leads to neuromuscular pain. Because it's harder to be as industrious, responsible, reliable, functional, and trustworthy as before and they seek favorable recognition, their anxiety worsens and pain increases. Several studies have shown that mild anxiety was present in 50–75% before the syn-drome was diagnosed.

Other personality profiles may be present. Up to 20% of university-based fibromyalgia patients may have post-traumatic stress disorder (PTSD, see below), 20% severe emotional neglect and/or abuse, 20% chronic depression and 5% panic disorders.

Post-Traumatic Stress Disorder (PTSD)

Increased pain levels, emotional distress, varying degrees of disability and interference with function are present in up to 20% of severe fibromyalgia patients at tertiary centers. Usually brought on by a specific traumatic event (e.g., death of a loved one), or continuous unpleasant circumstances (e.g., a tour of duty during the Afghan War), PTSD is associated with nightmares, recurrent and intensive recollections, fear, catastrophizing, and avoidance of thoughts and activities associated with the traumatic event or events. PTSD patients are easily aroused and display hypervigilance relating to fear and pain catastrophizing. They tend to be more aware of normal bodily sensa-tions such as perception or sensitivity to noises, light, and heartbeats, and frequently complain of dizziness. PTSD is more prevalent in patients who have a family history of sexual, physical, or verbal abuse, domestic violence, alcoholism or addiction.

ARE THERE OTHER DISORDERS THAT FIBROMYALGIA PATIENTS DO NOT HAVE AND THAT REQUIRE DIFFERENTIATION?

There are other conditions that some doctors confuse with fibromyalgia, and several surveys cited above show that patients generally do *not* have them. Some of these conditions are described below.

Hypochondriasis

Hypochondriacs have an excessive fear of having a serious disease based on misinterpretation of one or more bodily symptoms and signs. They believe normal bodily sensations such as heartbeats and peristalsis represent a medical disorder. Nearly all fibromyalgia patients want to get well and accept reassurance that they are not seriously ill.

Hysteria (Conversion Reactions)

The psychiatric definition of hysteria differs from the common perception that these are individuals who are prone to ranting or raving. Hysterical patients complain of neurologic or body deficits that are not real and display a lack of concern (*la belle indifference*) or act blase about them. These conversion reactions involve statements that they cannot see, hear, or talk, or are paralyzed. An example would be a soldier in battle who reports that he cannot move his legs. Some aspects of hysteria infrequently overlap with fibromyalgia, but hysteria is usually not associated with the syndrome.

Psychogenic Rheumatism

Patients who claim that they "hurt all over" but lack fibromyalgia tender points and have changing stories with inappropriate or inconsistent responses have a *fictitious disease* known as *psychogenic rheumatism*. These patients have serious emotional problems, and their complaints satisfy the psychological need for attention. Some are *psychotic,* or have lost touch with reality. Their stories make no biologic sense. The classic example is the patient who complains that "I hurt on the left side of my body, from the top of my head to the bottom of my toe." Anatomically, this is impossible since the nerve supply of these areas crosses the spinal cord at the neck and the head would hurt on the opposite side. Tender points are not found on examination, and no arthritis or muscle-focused therapies ever work. *Malingering,* or producing symptoms and signs for external gain, is not a feature of fibromyalgia.

Body Dysmorphic Disorder

Sometimes we encounter patients who are engrossed with themselves. They express excessive concern or fear of having a defect in appearance, a condition termed *body dysmorphic disorder*. These patients obsess over every blemish or bruise. Studies have shown no correlation between this behavior pattern and fibromyalgia.

Obsessive-Compulsive Behavior

Many doctors think that most fibromyalgia patients have perfectionistic tendencies. After all, many new fibromyalgia patients came to us with a neatly typed, detailed medical history and list of complaints. *Obsessive-compulsive personality disorder* consists of a preoccupation with orderliness, perfectionism, and mental and interpersonal control at the expense of flexibility, openness, and efficiency. The bottom line is that perfectionism as part of obsessive-compulsive personality disorder is not more common, but perfectionistic tendencies may be.

Bipolar Illness

Familial studies have also shown that patients with *bipolar illness (manic-depressive psychosis)* are at a 150-fold increased risk for developing FM. Bipolar illness affects 1% of the United States population, but may represent up to 10% of FM patients. As known as manic-depressive disorder, patients often describe severe pain but when undistracted have little in the way of an abnormal tender point examination. Their complaints are so convincing that demanding doctors "cut it out" or "remove it" leads to unnecessary imaging, procedures, nerve blocks, and surgical interventions. The treatment can be frustrating, as these patients respond poorly to musculoskeletal and pain directed interventions, and need specific medications that are used for this indication (e.g., a family known as "atypical antipsychotics"). In our opinoin, bipolar illness is a form of "pseudofibromyalgia".

SUMMING UP

As already noted, population-based studies have demonstrated that the relationship between pain and distress is complex and that distress is both a cause and consequence of pain. In this latter instance, a typical pattern is that as a result of pain and other symptoms of FM, individuals begin to function less well in their various roles. They may have difficulties with spouses, children, and work around the home, which exacerbate symptoms and lead to maladaptive illness behaviors. These include isolation, cessation of pleasurable activities, reductions in activity and exercise, etc. In the worst cases, patients become involved with disability and compensation systems, that almost ensure that they will not improve.

The complex interaction of biological, behavioral, psychological, and behavioral mechanisms is not, however, unique to FM. Non-biological factors play a prominent role in symptom expression in all rheumatic diseases. In fact, in conditions such as rheumatoid arthritis and osteoarthritis, non-biological factors such as level of formal education, coping strategies, and socioeconomic variables account for more of the variance in pain report and disability than biologic factors, such as the joint space width or sedimentation rate.

Because of the biopsychosocial nature of fibromyalgia, several groups have attempted to identify subgroups of individuals with this condition, that may present differently or respond differentially to treatment. One of these studies examined how differential degrees of depression, maladaptive cognitions, and hyperalgesia might interact to lead to different subgroups of patients.

Three identified subgroups can be usefully identified. The first comprises approximately half of the patients who have low levels of depression and anxiety, normal cognition regarding pain, and are mildly tender (although tender enough to meet the ACR criteria). The second subgroup, representative of a "tertiary care" fibromyalgia patient, are slightly more tender, and also displayed high levels of depression. These patients also have cognitions associated with a poor prognosis in many pain conditions. These include an external locus of pain control, defined as feeling that they can do nothing about their pain, and catastrophizing, defined as having a very negative and pessimistic view of their pain. The third subgroup, perhaps the most interesting, are the most tender, but with no negative psychological or cognitive factors. This suggests that in some "resilient" individuals, positive psychological and cognitive factors issues may actually "buffer" neurobiological factors leading to pain and other symptoms in FM.

Patients with fibromyalgia are not crazy and are infrequently depressed. They tend to experience more psychological distress, mild chronic anxiety, and psychosocial disruption. These manifestations are often associated with perfectionistic tendencies and hypervigilance of normal bodily sensations. A biomedical model, wherein a biologic or physiologic response to pain influences psychologic well-being, is the appropriate way to view fibromyalgia.

FOR FURTHER READING

Gupta A, Silman AJ, Ray D, *et al.* The role of psychosocial factors in predicting the onset of chronic widespread pain: Results from a prospective population-based study, *Rheumatology* 2007; *46*: 666–671.

Hauser W, Kosseva M, Uceyler N, *et al*. Emotional, physical and sexual abuse in fibromyalgia syndrome: A systemic review with meta-analysis. *Arthritis Care Res* 2011; *63*: 808–820.

Hudson JI, Goldenberg DL, Pope HG., *et al*. Comorbidity of fibromyalgia with medical and psychiatric disorders. *Amer J Med 92*, 1992: 363–367.

McBeth J, Macfarlane GJ, Benjamin S, Silman AJ. Features of somatization predict the onset of chronic widespread pain. *Arthritis Rheum 44*, 2001: 940–946.

Taylor ML, Trotter DR, Csuka ME. The prevalence of sexual abuse in women with fibromyalgia. *Arthritis Rheum 38*, 1995: 229–234.

Wallace DJ, Clauw DJ, Hallegua DS. Addressing behavioral abnormalities in fibromyalgia. *J Musculoskeletal Med* 2005: 22: 562–579.

Wallace DJ, Gotto J. Hypothesis: Bipolar illness with complaints of chronic musculoskeletal pain is a form of pseudofibromyalgia, *Semin Arthritis Rheum* 2008; *37*: 256–259.

Part VI
IMPROVING YOUR QUALITY OF LIFE

Based on our experience, fewer than half of the six million Americans with fibromyalgia are taking prescription medication for complaints related to the syndrome. How do they get by? Whether or not formally diagnosed with fibromyalgia, these individuals (as well as those who take medication) instinctively make changes in their lifestyle. However, the quest for an improved quality of life is paved with uncertainties and unproven approaches. The next three chapters review how the symptoms and signs of fibromyalgia are influenced by daily activities and explore how approaches to diet, exercise, and personal interactions allow fibromyalgia patients to live a productive and fulfilling life.

18

Influences of Lifestyle and Environment on Fibromyalgia

A man cannot be comfortable without his own approval.
> Mark Twain (1835–1910),
> *What Is Man?* (1906)

Although there is no cure for fibromyalgia, patients can initiate numerous changes and make adjustments that improve their sense of well being. Simply stated, there are things patients can do without spending money or seeing a health care provider. Demonstrating a certain amount of control over the syndrome also improves self-esteem and instills a sense of self-worth.

This chapter describes how modifications in diet, sleep habits, and lifestyle can ameliorate fibromyalgia. It also advises patients how best to deal with the weather, fatigue, pain, and their home environment so that they will hurt less and become more productive.

VITAMINS AND FOOD FOR THOUGHT: IS THERE A FIBROMYALGIA DIET?

What some call health, if purchased by perpetual anxiety about diet, isn't much better than tedious disease.
> George Dennison Prentice (1802–1870),
> *Prenticeana*, 1860

Even though certain general dietary principles allow fibromyalgia patients to feel better, there is no "fibromyalgia diet." No specific food regimens or supplements have ever been shown in any published, controlled study to be helpful for fibromyalgia despite the observation that "arthritis diet" books are a multi-million-dollar-a-year industry.

How can we explain this discrepancy? First, people feel better when they eat healthy foods. Most "arthritis diet" books urge patients to eat three well-balanced meals a day and caution against overeating. Many recommend having the main meal at midday; heavy, late-evening dinners don't give the body enough time to burn off calories and are associated with bedtime esophageal spasm or heartburn.

Similarly, consuming alcohol, nicotine, or caffeine (in the form of coffee, tea, or even chocolate) at a late dinner can make it harder to get a good night's sleep. Alcohol, in particular, should not be used as a painkiller. In turn, poor sleep can increase musculoskeletal pain. An acceptable healthy balance of proteins, carbohydrates, and fats can also increase energy and fight fatigue.

What about vitamins? As people always on the go, Americans tend to settle for the convenience of quick-to-prepare, easy-to-consume refined, processed foods that are relatively deficient in vitamins and minerals. Multivitamin and mineral supplements can be useful additions for those who don't have time or are unable to prepare well-balanced meals. Many specialized formulas with heavily promoted "herbs and spices" are available from acquaintances, distributors, and health food stores; none of these have been shown to be superior to Wal-Mart, Rite-Aid, or CVS preparations available at a fraction of the cost. Most vitamins, herbs, minerals, and supplements added to multivitamins are harmless, but some are occasionally associated with allergic reactions (see Chapter 23).

Food sensitivity plays a role in less than 10% of our fibromyalgia patients. Within this group, different foods affect people differently. For example, some fibromyalgia patients feel better when they eat fish, while others hurt more. Some practitioners believe that carbohydrates increase serotonin levels, essential fatty acids diminish fatigue, and proteins improve mental alertness. Others place patients on a hypoglycemic/yeast elimination diet consisting of small, frequent meals, along with carbohydrate and wheat product restrictions. A few patients have had success with the Dong arthritis diet, a Duke University elimination diet that recognizes individual food sensitivity differences and provides a means for investigating what one can or cannot tolerate. We neither endorse nor refute any diet or food regimen for fibromyalgia, since none have been studied in a scientifically acceptable fashion. Thus, we have no admonitions for fibromyalgia patients regarding specific food groups.

BONING UP: DOES FIBROMYALGIA INTERACT WITH BONE DEMINERALIZATION?

As we age, our bones lose calcium. The loss of calcium leads to the thinning of our bony architecture and affects its structural integrity. When bone mineralization decreases to a specified level, the consequences may lead to fracture. In the United States, 25 million Americans have *osteoporosis* (or very thin bones), which is associated with 1.3 million fractures annually. Twenty percent of these fractures rob patients of the ability to live independently for varying periods of time, which results in pain management problems and loss of self-esteem.

The overwhelming majority of patients with osteoporosis are females, most of whom are menopausal. Although fibromyalgia does not cause or accelerate osteoporosis, it indirectly influences the disorder. For instance, exercise and other forms of physical activity help prevent calcium loss from the bone, while smoking, poor nutrition, immobilization, and inactivity promote it. If fibromyalgia

Table 18.1. *Calcium supplementation*

---

1. Foods with high calcium content (the average U.S. diet contains 600 mg a day)

Milk, 8 oz, 300 mg	Hard cheese, 1 oz, 200 mg
Ice cream, 1 cup, 176 mg	Oysters, 1/2 cup, raw, 113 mg
Broccoli, 1 cup, 136 mg	Sardines, canned, 3 oz, 372 mg
One large orange, 78 mg	Spinach, 1/2 cup, raw, 111 mg
Yogurt, 8 oz, 400 mg	

2. Oral calcium supplements including examples of calcium products. Never take in over 600 mg at a time. The body does not absorb more. Reserve some calcium for bedtime.

Calcium carbonate: OsCal, Turns, Titralac, Maalox, Mylanta

Calcium citrate: Citrical, Caltrate

Calcium gluconate: Calcet

Calcium lactate: store brands

3. Vitamin D improves the absorption of calcium by the gastrointestinal tract. The easiest way to derive enough vitamin D is by taking 2000 u daily.

---

patients carry out the physical measures reviewed in Chapter 19, their risk of developing osteoporosis diminishes. From a dietary standpoint it appears prudent to increase calcium in the diet or to supplement meals with at least 1.0 to 1.5 grams of calcium a day. Table 18.1 lists several ways this can be accomplished.

ARE THERE MORE REASONS WHY SMOKING IS BAD?

Don't smoke. It's not only bad for obvious reasons, it also aggravates fibromyalgia. Nicotine is a stimulant, which can make it harder to sleep at night. Cigarettes induce hyperreactivity in airways in the lung, cause wheezing, and decrease stamina. Over time, smoking accelerates atherosclerosis, or hardening of the arteries, which diminishes the amount of oxygen delivered to muscles; this, in turn, can cause pain. Dr. Yunus at the University of Illinois (Peoria) has demonstrated that smokers with fibromyalgia have lower pain thresholds and more sleep problems than nonsmokers. Nicotine withdrawal has been associated with muscle spasms. Finally, vascular constriction or spasm caused by abnormal functioning of the ANS (see Chapter 7), observed in 30–40% of fibromyalgia patients, is worsened by smoking and leads to increased numbness, burning, and tingling.

In other words, there are absolutely no healthy reasons to smoke!

CAN FIBROMYALGIA BE BLAMED ON THE WEATHER?

Sunshine is delicious, rain is refreshing, wind braces us, snow is exhilarating; there is no such thing as bad weather, only different kinds of weather.
                                                    John Ruskin (1819–1900)

There is no question about it, nearly all patients feel that climate influences their fibromyalgia. In one survey, 66% of fibromyalgia patients related that they were affected by weather changes: 78% preferred warm weather, 79% believed that cold weather made them feel worse, and 60% did not like humidity. A variety of studies have suggested that musculoskeletal stiffness, achiness, and pain are aggravated by *changes* in barometric pressure. Fibromyalgia symptoms can be aggravated when the weather shifts from hot to cold or from wet to dry. A consistent climate is associated with fewer musculoskeletal symptoms. For instance, Hawaii theoretically has the perfect climate for fibromyalgia patients since it is usually within four degrees of 83°F and humid year round. However, before contacting a realtor, it's important to realize that this does not allow for changes in barometric pressure from walking into and out of air-conditioned buildings all day. What's the best way to deal with changes in climate? Don't panic or get upset if it takes a few days to acclimatize when traveling or if the weather changes.

Fibromyalgia patients living in northern climates are especially susceptible to a condition known as *seasonal affective disorder.* Light deprivation during the winter predisposes one to depression and fatigue. This can lead to decreased energy, productivity, motivation, libido, patience, and the ability to focus one's thoughts. Bright lights or a midwinter trip to Southern California, Arizona, or Florida can help break this form of emotional paralysis.

BUT I'M SO TIRED!

The feeling of sleepiness when you are not in bed and can't get there, is the meanest feeling in the world.

Edgar Watson Howe (1853–1937),
Country Town Sayings, 1911

Fatigue is a significant complaint in 75–80% of fibromyalgia patients. It can destroy relationships, lower self-esteem, and cause other people to accuse one of "making it up" since fibromyalgia patients generally look healthy. There are many things that can be done before considering medication. Once other medical problems that cause fatigue are ruled out, there are better ways to manage daily activities.

First, is the patient taking prescription medications (especially muscle relaxants) during the day that make them tired? Can alcohol or illicit drug use be a factor? The fibromyalgia patient should avoid daytime napping after the early afternoon; otherwise it's harder to sleep at night. Many patients have overextended lives and, before becoming ill, were intensely active, and overinvolved perfectionistic (but not obsessive) tendencies also can lead to fatigue since these individuals push to accomplish more than they are really able to do. It's important to establish realistic goals.

Here are a few tips on how to overcome fatigue. Most important, learn the concept of pacing. Be busy for a couple of hours in the morning and then take a 15- to 20-minute break. Engage in activities for another two hours and eat a leisurely lunch. Alternating periods of activity with rest times allow most fibromyalgia patients to be as productive as healthy people. Don't stay in bed all day trying to conserve energy. This can lead to depression, premature osteoporosis, atrophy of the muscles, flexion contractures, and *increased* pain over time because poor conditioning prevents muscles from getting enough oxygen.

If fatigue is an overwhelming problem, adopt a strategy to deal with it. First, get a good night's sleep and embark on a conditioning program. Plan ahead and try to accomplish only what is really important. Learn to have certain responsibilities handled by others and limit commitments. Within the confines of the pacing concept, learn to manage time, use energy wisely, and perform tasks requiring the greatest amount of focusing and energy at the time of day when functioning best. Many fibromyalgia patients have a midday "window" of feeling better—for example, from 10 A.M. to 2 P.M. Sometimes medications are given to decrease fatigue; these are reviewed in Chapter 22. Remember, there are many things that alleviate fatigue short of taking medicine.

I DON'T SLEEP WELL!

That we are not much sicker and much madder than we are is due exclusively to that most blessed and blessing of all natural graces, sleep.
Aldous Huxley (1894–1963),
Variations on a Philosopher, 1950

A good night's sleep is critical to overcoming fibromyalgia. Sleep heals our muscles and decreases daytime fatigue. Over 75% of fibromyalgia patients report significant sleep problems. The presentations of sleep complaints and a discussion of the biology of sleep in fibromyalgia were reviewed in Chapters 6 and 10.

Before considering a prescription sleep aid, there are many things that can be done to improve the sleep environment. First, take a look at the bedroom. Is the bed comfortable, the mattress firm, and the pillows suitable? A cervical pillow reduces neck strain because it is shaped to support the neck. The room should be quiet and comfortable in temperature with a climate control system that keeps it neither too hot nor too cold. Don't let pets into the bedroom. Don't sleep with children. Don't exercise vigorously after dinner. And allow the room to become dark before going to bed.

Start preparing for a good night's sleep early in the day. Have a regular bedtime and wake-up time. Don't nap after early afternoon. Don't drink a lot of fluids or take diuretics in the evening. Avoid caffeine, tobacco, alcohol, or a spicy or large meal too close to bedtime. On the other hand, don't starve, since hunger can also interfere with sleep. Use the hour before lights out to prepare for sleep. Think pleasing thoughts and practice slow, deep breathing. Soft music or relaxation tapes promote a restful mindset. Soak in a hot tub or take a hot shower and mentally close the day. Try not to read or listen to anything disturbing.

When the lights are turned out, one should fall asleep in 15–20 minutes. Falling asleep in less than five minutes suggests a state of sleep deprivation; on the other hand, if 30 minutes have elapsed, get up, since it's not time to sleep. With fibromyalgia, pain can make it difficult to fall or stay asleep, and patients need all the help they can muster. It may be more comfortable to lie on the back or side, or place a pillow under the knees to ease pressure on the lower back. If it's cold, consider using an extra blanket.

Once asleep, try to sleep enough to feel refreshed in the morning. Make sure bed partners do not snore to the point of interfering with needed rest. Don't keep the television or radio on. If you awaken at 3 A.M. and cannot sleep, get up and putter. The problem should take care of itself within a few nights.

These routines are inexpensive and easy to carry out. Many fibromyalgia patients can overcome sleep problems without medication if they focus attention on their sleep environment.

DOCTOR, I'M IN PAIN!

An hour of pain is as long as a day of pleasure.

English proverb

Pain is a natural sensation that is an unavoidable feature of fibromyalgia. Don't let it be controlling—learn to control it. In pain amplification syndromes such as fibromyalgia, distractions make us less aware of discomfort. Whether we are listening to music, driving a car, watching a movie, or performing work activities, pain perception is lessened when we don't concentrate on it. Biofeedback, meditation, and other techniques reviewed in Chapter 19 help send healing messages to painful areas. Fibromyalgia pain is never caused by and does not lead to crippling deformities. It's impossible to hurt yourself while "walking through the pain" by sublimating the sensation.

MAKING A HOUSE A HOME

Fibromyalgia may try to control the patient, but one way of fighting back is to create a home environment that minimizes the opportunity of producing discomfort. A little thought and organization can greatly improve the way one feels. In turn, this decreases pain without sapping precious energy reserves.

How can this be accomplished? Consolidate and simplify household chores—cook for two meals at once, take breaks, and perform only simple tasks when energy levels are low. Arrange activities to decrease the times needed to walk up and down stairs. Avoid putting things that get a lot of use in high cupboards and cabinets should have large handles for grasping. Rolling carts offer accessible, additional workspace. Use felt marker pens, which put less stress on the hands, and don't write for long periods of time. Of all the regular household activities, vacuuming is the worst. A vacuum cleaner's use aggravates back, shoulder, and arm discomfort and produces pain more often than any other appliance. Break up the activity. For starters, buy a lightweight vacuum cleaner and don't try to vacuum the whole house at once. When washing dishes, distribute body weight with one foot on a stepstool and try not to lean too far forward. Similarly, put one foot on a footstool while ironing to reduce back strain. When washing windows, dusting, or scrubbing, find devices with longer, larger handles. If necessary, have somebody help carry in the groceries. Make your house more user-friendly. If appropriate, put grab bars in the bathroom, change front door handles to levers, raise electrical outlets and phone jacks to a higher level, buy nonskid rugs, and use pullout drawers or Lazy Susans.

Time and energy are too precious to squander...and this is one area where fibromyalgia patients have a lot of control.

AUTOMOBILES AND TRAVELING

It's important to get out and around, and most fibromyalgia patients travel in a car. Body mechanics in an automobile can make things better or worse. Bucket seats are more comfortable than bench seats. Make sure that the seat is adjustable and has armrests. The ideal vehicle for fibromyalgia patients should have an adequate headrest at the middle of the head for support, a climate control system, and automatic transmission. Mirrors should be plentiful, well-placed, and easy to adjust. Don't recline, slouch, or sit too close to the steering column. For those with low back problems, buying a lumbar cushion accessory may be useful.

While on vacation, take plenty of breaks from driving or sightseeing, find a flexible travel partner, and get a good night's sleep. Some fibromyalgia patients bring their own neck collars or pillows with them. Don't be shy about using special luggage racks, carts, or wheels. Don't let isolation creep into your life—go out, travel, and enjoy!

HOW DO INFECTIONS INFLUENCE FIBROMYALGIA?

Most fibromyalgia patients have a normal immune system and don't get colds or other infections more frequently than other people. However, infections can aggravate fibromyalgia symptoms, and patients often take longer to recover. For example, when fibromyalgia patients develop bronchitis, persistent coughing frequently intensifies myofascial pain in the upper back. Fevers decrease stamina to a greater extent than in a healthy person. Viruses can lead to temporary relapses of fatigue syndromes. It's important to cope with these frustrations in a productive way. Some fibromyalgia patients need to pace themselves and take it a bit more slowly than usual for a little longer.

SUMMING UP

Certain aspects of life can be easily controlled. Fibromyalgia's impact can be reduced by eating a healthy, well-balanced diet with appropriate vitamin and mineral supplements when needed, not smoking, minimizing the effects of changes in barometric pressure, pacing, managing time, getting a good night's sleep, and creating a home and travel environment that decreases activities known to produce fatigue, pain, and strain. The measures reviewed in this chapter are inexpensive, practical, and don't require visits to health care professionals.

FOR FURTHER READING

Burckhardt CS. Nonpharmacological management strategies in fibromyalgia. *Rheum Dis North America* 2002; *28*: 291–304.

Pellegrino M. *Inside Fibromyalgia. Columbus*, Ohio: Anadem Publishing, 2001.

19

The Influence of Exercise and Rehabilitation on the Mind and Body

We are under-exercised as a nation. We look instead of play. We ride instead of walk. Our existence deprives us of the minimum of physical activity essential for healthy living.

John F. Kennedy (1917–1963)

Let's continue on the self-help road to improving fibromyalgia symptoms. Suppose we are eating healthy, well-balanced meals, are no longer smoking, have learned to pace ourselves, cope with changes in the weather, are sleeping well, and have reconfigured the house. At this point, how can the body be trained to reduce pain, stiffness, and fatigue? This chapter will explore how physical, mental, and complementary modalities allow fibromyalgia patients to feel better about their bodies and minds.

PRINCIPLES OF FIBROMYALGIA REHABILITATION

Therapeutic regimens that help the body and mind, whether physical therapy, pilates, yoga, acupuncture, or chiropractic methods, are all based on similar tenets of body mechanics:

1. Fibromyalgia patients will never improve unless they have good posture. Bad posture aggravates musculoskeletal pain and creates tight, stiff, sore muscles. Therefore, stretch, change positions, and have a good workstation that does not require too much leaning or reaching.
2. The way we get around is a demonstration of body mechanics. The fundamental principles of good body mechanics in fibromyalgia include using a broad base of support by distributing loads to stronger joints with a greater surface area, keeping things close to the body to provide leverage, minimizing reaching, and not putting too much pressure on the lower back (demonstrated in Figure 21). Also, don't stay in the same position for a prolonged period of time.

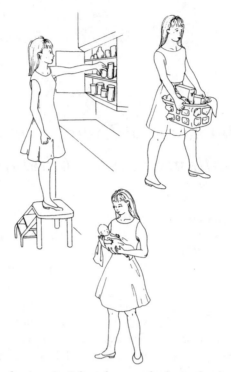

Fig. 19.1. *The basic principles of proper body mechanics that enhance well-being in fibromyalgia.*

3. Exercise is necessary. It improves our sense of well-being, strengthens muscles and bones, allows restful sleep, relieves stress, releases serotonin and endorphins, which decreases pain, and burns calories.
4. Don't be shy about using supports. Whether it be an armrest, special chair, brace, wall, railing, pillow, furniture, slings, pockets, or even another person's body, supports allow fibromyalgia patients to decrease the amount of weight or stress that would otherwise be applied to the body, producing discomfort or pain.
5. All activities should be conducive to relaxation and stress reduction, whether they be deep breathing, meditation, biofeedback, or guided imagery.

There are a surprisingly large number of ways these activities can be carried out. They are discussed in the next few sections. See Figure 19.1.

PHYSICAL MODALITIES

The traditional methods for strengthening muscles, improving body mechanics and posture, and preventing damage are through exercise, physical therapy, and occupational therapy.

Why Does Exercise Hurt Me More?

Many patients with fibromyalgia were physically quite vigorous before they developed the syndrome. A common complaint is that when they tried to resume their activities, exercise only increased their exhaustion and pain. One survey showed that 83% of fibromyalgia patients do not exercise regularly and 80% are not considered physically fit. Some of the more common aggravating activities include heavy lifting or pulling. The CDC has even included "postexertion malaise" as a criterion for defining chronic fatigue syndrome. How can this paradox be explained?

As reviewed in Chapters 4–7, pain can result when muscles don't get enough oxygen. A consequence of changes in the ANS's signals is that this lack of oxygen and inefficient utilization of oxygen is further compounded by excessive constriction of blood vessels. In other words, when a fibromyalgia patient tries to exercise, a vicious cycle is unleashed. When blood vessels don't allow enough oxygen to be delivered to muscle tissue, even mild exercise produces microtrauma, or "angina," in muscles and pain. Further, microtrauma to the muscles can't be repaired at night since not enough growth hormone is released when we sleep poorly. In turn, these factors lead patients to avoid exercise in order to minimize discomfort. Over time, muscle atrophy, or wasting, and osteoporosis, or thinning of the bones, develop. This limits the patient's reserves and produces deconditioning so that even mild exertion results in profound fatigue.

What Is the Best Kind of Exercise for Fibromyalgia?

How can fibromyalgia patients overcome the vicious cycle of exercise-pain-fatigue-exercise-pain-fatigue? First, motivation to undertake a gradual, progressive course of increasing activity and exercise is important. Try walking as the initial activity. Walk for five minutes twice a day, increasing to 45 minutes. Take breaks or sit on a bench if this makes you feel fatigued or winded. Walking is the first step toward a general conditioning and toning program. It diminishes stiffness. Over time, it relieves muscle and vascular spasm and allows more oxygen to reach the tissues. If the weather is bad, walk in an indoor mall. Walking with a friend can take the mind off what's going on, and time passes more easily.

Gradually, other general conditioning programs such as swimming and bicycling can be added to the regimen. Swimming for 30 to 60 minutes three times a week is an excellent way to strengthen muscles and condition the body. The buoyancy of water moves joints through their full range of motion and strengthens muscles with less stress, as you move in ways that are difficult outside of water. Swimmers bear only 10% of their body weight. While swimming, increased chest expansion allows for deeper breathing and more oxygen being taken in. Bicycling is an excellent activity that promotes general conditioning.

Before buying a bicycle (stationary or otherwise), try it out and make sure the seat, handlebars, and amount of pedal resistance are comfortable.

Exercises are divided into several categories. In their simplest form, *isometric* exercises are useful in fibromyalgia. These routines allow patients to build muscle strength without moving, permitting a muscle to stretch until tension is felt. For example, the strap muscles in the neck can be strengthened by a cervical isometric program. If a patient pushes the forehead with moderate force against the hand placed against it and holds it for six seconds, the sustained muscle contraction (if repeated two times, twice a day along with other maneuvers as shown in Figure 19.2) will strengthen the neck. This, in turn, protects patients against maneuvers, lurches, or sprains that increase upper back and lower neck strain. Along with isometric exercises, physical therapists frequently add *stretching* exercises to the regimen. Stretching (Pilates is an excellent example) does not allow jerking or bouncing around, decreases muscle tightness, prevents spasm, and is performed together with deep-breathing exercises. Fibromyalgia patients often have shallow, jerky breathing patterns; slow, deep, rhythmic breathing promotes energy and allows relaxation.

Over time, patients work their way up to *isotonic* exercises that start with low-impact aerobics, where at least one foot is on the floor and there is no jumping. In their most helpful form, after a warmup period these activities allow enough arm and body movement to increase the heart rate without producing a jarring sensation that often makes fibromyalgia worse. We encourage

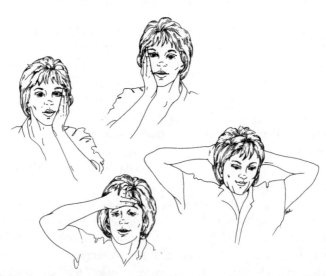

Fig. 19.2. *An example of strength-building isometric exercises. Performing these four cervical isometric maneuvers as sustained contractions for 6 seconds, twice a day, morning and evening, strengthens the sternocleidomastoid muscles and makes the neck less vulnerable to pain after injury or trauma.*

fibromyalgia patients not to place too much tension on tender areas and have found that pain is accentuated by weight lifting, rowing, jogging, or playing tennis, golf, or bowling early in the course of rehabilitation. Isotonic exercises are not for everybody and should be built up slowly. Make sure that a physician approves of the amount of exertion involved in an exercise program from a cardiovascular standpoint.

Aerobic exercises are designed to increase oxygen consumption by increasing the heart rate and are useful later on.

How Can a Physical Therapist Help Fibromyalgia?

Physical therapists are health care professionals who usually have had four to six years of formal education after high school. They help patients achieve physical conditioning by using several modalities, especially the sorts of exercises reviewed above. Some additional modalities are the following:

1. *Massage* allows deep muscles to relax, loosens tight muscles, relieves pain and spasm, improves circulation, and decreases stress. Massages should be gentle so as not to aggravate fibromyalgia symptoms. The Alexander technique emphasizes posture and movement along with massage, and the Feldenkreis method incorporates massage with body-mind communication enhancements.
2. *Spray and stretch* is a technique by which a cool spray (ethyl chloride or fluorimethane) is applied to a painful area, numbing the nerves locally, and is followed by gentle stretching of the muscle underneath it, promoting relaxation.
3. *Heat* relaxes muscles and can be applied with the use of blankets, showers, waterbeds, hot tubs, lamps, microwave gelpacks, heating pads, or a hydroculator. Moist heat is usually more effective than dry heat. Therapists frequently use ultrasound to deliver deep heat to painful areas in a relaxing, rhythmic motion. These sound waves go to the muscles, tendons, and soft tissues. A variant of this technique is iontophoresis, in which medication such as xylocaine or a local steroid can be administered to painful areas. Temperatures above 90°F (such as in a jacuzzi or hot tub) should not be applied to any area of the body for longer than 15 minutes since the treatment can produce lightheadedness, dizziness, low blood pressure, or excessive fatigue.
4. *Ice* or cold packs treat injuries or strains less than 36 hours old by decreasing swelling. Approximately 15% of our fibromyalgia patients prefer cold to heat and benefit from ice massages. Icing an area for 10-15 minutes before vigorous activity (e.g., the shoulder before playing tennis or the shins prior to jogging) minimizes postexertional muscle pain in patients who are deconditioned.

5. *Electrical stimulation* delivers electrical impulses to nerves that, in turn block painful messages. A form of electronic acupuncture, this can be accomplished by a TENS unit, acuscope, neuroprobe, or muscle exerciser.

6. Although chiropractors and osteopaths are known for their *manipulation* techniques, physical therapists also use traction, manipulation, and myo-fascial release.

7. *Posture and gait training* involves watching how patients walk and "carry" themselves. After evaluating a patient's body mechanics, the therapist may recommend strengthening and range-of-motion exercises, or assistive devices such as splints, collars, or braces.

8. The choice of *footwear* used while exercising or for everyday use is impor-tant. For the latter, the least expensive and most comfortable daily shoe is a sneaker a half size too big. For exercise, there should be no pressure on the sides or toe tips, heel counters should hold the heel firmly, and the shoe should be comfortable. Shoes with widened toe areas or Velcro straps rather than laces may be desirable.

9. Physical therapists often work with occupational therapists or counselors to assist patients with *relaxation techniques.* These include biofeedback, deep-breathing exercises, guided imagery, and meditation.

If you are getting physical therapy at a large institution, try to see the same therapist each time. Camaraderie and close working relationships are associated with better outcomes.

What Is an Occupational Therapist?

The term *occupational therapist* is very misleading. Vocational rehabilitation counselors, not occupational therapists, advise patients about what employment is best for them and arrange for appropriate coursework and training. Occupational therapists practice a discipline known as *ergonomics* in designing work tasks to fit the capabilities of the human body (see Chapter 24). They perform an ADL, or Activities of Daily Living evaluation. Occupational therapists consider such questions as: How much energy do people waste performing various chores such as housework? Is there a better way to get into and out of a car, on and off a toilet seat, or into and out of a bathtub? Occupational therapists apply prin-ciples of energy conservation and joint protection in their evaluations. Many large companies have therapists on site to evaluate workstations, office furniture, com-puter screen levels, and distances. Is the office environment smoke-free, aestheti-cally pleasing, and user-friendly? (See Chapter 24.) Is there adaptive equipment such as a longer or thicker handle that decreases reaching, bending, or lifting? Is splinting or bracing useful? Occupational therapists are experts when it comes to using or designing special wheels, levers, lightweight objects, enlarged handles, or specialized convenience tools. In our opinion, these underutilized professionals are unsung heroes responsible for a portion of the increased corporate productivity that the United States has enjoyed over the last 20 years.

When Is a Physical Or Occupational Therapy Evaluation Useful?

In our experience, patients with mild fibromyalgia infrequently need a formal rehabilitation program. Many physical therapists have little training concerning the needs of fibromyalgia patients and should consider taking a course the Arthritis Foundation offers to be up-to-date. Unfortunately, only one-third of our patients tell us that physical therapy was very useful, one-third report that they felt fine for a few hours afterward before returning to their baseline condition, and one-third say that they felt worse because the program was too aggressive or hard on the soft tissues. In the hands of highly proficient physical and occupational therapists, chronically ill patients or those refractory to treatment can have dramatic responses to a well-designed, well-thought-out rehabilitation program. An outstanding example with a high published success rate is the program devised by Drs. Sharon Clark and Robert Bennett at the University of Oregon Heath Sciences Center in Portland.

We usually prescribe physical and occupational therapy in tandem with medication to our patients who perform moderate to severe activity. The ideal program consists of 12 to16 45-minute sessions over three to four months, after which patients can exercise independently and do their own rehabilitation. Most insurance carriers will pay for 10 to 20 physical therapy sessions a year if the need is well documented. About 10% of our fibromyalgia patients, especially those with reflex sympathetic dystrophy, benefit from one or two years of physical therapy.

MENTAL MODALITIES

Anybody who is 25 or 30 years old has physical scars from all sorts of things, from tuberculosis to polio. It's all the same with the mind.
                    Ralph Kaufman, 20th century health practitioner

Mental health professionals have become increasingly interested in using their expertise and resources to help fibromyalgia patients. *Psychiatrists* are medical doctors and can prescribe medication. *Psychologists* have a master's degree or a doctorate, are not physicians, and cannot prescribe medication. *Medical or psychiatric social workers* frequently work with psychologists and psychiatrists and provide counseling services. Some *nurse practitioners* or *physician's assistants* have specialized psychiatric training. Members of the *clergy* frequently fulfill a healing role in advising and assisting fibromyalgia patients. Most have some training, and many have degrees in psychology, counseling, or social work. Traditionally, these health professionals use a variety of techniques to decrease stress, enhance coping skills, diminish fatigue, build self-esteem, and improve interpersonal interactions. Patients must feel comfortable with their therapists, and there should be a minimum of distraction during therapy sessions.

Classical Psychotherapy

We refer 10–20% of our fibromyalgia patients to psychotherapists. Fibromyalgia patients who are the best candidates for classical psychotherapy are in touch with reality and capable of having stable relationships with people, looking at themselves realistically, and being introspective. They should be willing to accept personal responsibility, have no secondary gain from their symptoms, and be interested in learning how to deal with anxiety, anger, or frustration without "acting out." The goals of therapy sessions are to verbalize concerns, confront inappropriate behavior patterns, clarify or understand these patterns based on past experiences, and work through problems. Patients should be able to identify their fears and destructive thinking patterns. They should try not to blame or make broad judgments. The treating professional and patient must form a therapeutic alliance enabling patients to develop a constructive means for dealing with problems that are prolonging stress, fatigue, or pain.

Cognitive Therapy: An Approach to "Brain Fatigue"

Cognitive therapy is a useful approach for patients with fibromyalgia who have difficulty learning, retaining, processing, recalling, finding words, focusing, concentrating, planning, or organizing. Cognitive dysfunction or impairment is usually intermittent and probably reflects spasm of blood vessels supplying oxygen to the brain as part of a dysfunctioning ANS (see Chapter 7). Most patients who report cognitive symptoms note that they are intermittent and of short duration. However, up to 10% of our patients have had to alter their lifestyle to accommodate cognitive symptoms. Cognitive behavioral interventions work to improve sleep, inactivity, and ANS awareness with the goal of increasing function, as well as decreasing fatigue, anxiety, and pain. Modalities used by therapists include simple relaxation, exercise, biofeedback, and spiritual counseling. Patients are educated about treating pain with nonprescription approaches.

Cognitive therapists usually are psychologists, occupational therapists, or speech therapists. They urge their clients to use memory aids such as placing project lists and Post-its around the house, decrease distractions, not to catastrophize, form mental pictures to assist with associations, and not to get frustrated when trying to find words. Bad moods, depression, and anxiety can have a negative influence on memory. Therapists show patients how to use cues, designate one spot at home as the repository of all knowledge, and write things down so that they will not forget. Having regular daily routines, using timers or alarm clocks, and having a regular filing system also are useful. Be frank about the problem; covering up "brain fatigue" only makes things worse.

Biofeedback and Stress-Reduction Strategies

Biofeedback works with making normally unconscious bodily actions conscious and controlling them to achieve relaxation and pain relief. Relaxation decreases SNS activity, slows the heart rate, and improves oxygen delivery to the muscles and brain. In particular, fibromyalgia patients have a heightened awareness of their autonomic functions such as pulse, blood pressure, and muscle tone. Electrical monitors can record skin temperature, heart rate, brain waves, digestion, and electrical skin conductivity (which measures muscle tension and is termed *EMG biofeedback*). Although at first glance it may seem like hocus-pocus, study after study has shown that deep-breathing exercises, relaxation tapes, and visualizing pleasant environments (called *guided imagery*) promote endorphin release and decrease muscle tension, pain, and stress. *EEG biofeedback* blocks some types of brain waves and reinforces others to improve cognitive, perceptual, and sleeping skills. For example, an EEG, or quantitative EEG can measure the frequencies of alpha (idling), beta (alert), theta (awake but drowsy), and delta (sleep) waves. Patients are trained to increase their beta waves. Stimulation with *cranial electrotherapy* can improve sleep and decrease pain. Biofeedback can be administered by physicians, physical therapists, occupational therapists, or psychologists, and is usually covered by insurance if the need for it is well documented.

Several controlled studies have shown that *cognitive behavioral therapy* improves fibromyalgia. These programs combine education, cognitive behavioral intervention, stress reduction techniques, support for family members and spouses, and strategies to improve physical fitness and flexibility. Biofeedback incorporates meditation, as do other techniques. For example, *yoga* combines deep breathing, meditation, and specific postures that integrate mental, physical, and spiritual energies to enhance well-being. *Transcendental meditation* enables patients to focus on a single thought or object to create an inner calm that banishes stress. *Tai chi* adds passive movements to achieve this result. Also, never underestimate the power of *prayer* along with quiet contemplation.

COMPLEMENTARY MODALITIES (ALTERNATIVE THERAPIES)

Formerly known as *alternative medicine,* complementary medicine approaches are defined as nontraditional therapeutic approaches practiced by physicians or health care professionals. In general, very few of these disciplines are taught in conventional medical schools. Why should we bother talking about complementary therapies? Simply because mainstream practitioners do not have all the answers, and some patients improve with these interventions. Why else would the U.S. public spend over $20 billion a year on complementary therapies, out of their own pockets? While some complementary modalities such as chiropractic are widely used and well established, others clearly have no place in managing fibromyalgia. This section will review some of these modalities. Homeopathy is covered in Chapter 23, and some complementary meditation techniques were reviewed in the previous section.

Does Acupuncture Work?

According to ancient Chinese tradition, yin and yang are complementary aspects of chi, an energizing life-force energy. Chi flows in the body through meridians, or imaginary lines along which the principles of acupuncture are based. Fine gauge, sterilized needles are inserted along these meridians to allow "energy paths" signaling the brain to heal pain. Used for over 2,500 years, acupuncture ideally should stimulate endorphin release and diminish pain in fibromyalgia tender points. In our experience, acupuncture is safe and inexpensive. TENS units and dry needling stimulate A-delta fibers, which diminishes pain by promoting the release of endorphins. The use of electrical acupuncture (see the physical therapy section of this chapter) is not restricted to the traditional meridians in relieving tender point pain. Most rheumatologists and published studies find the results of traditional acupuncture to be modest at best in managing fibromyalgia.

How Do Osteopaths Treat Fibromyalgia?

The discipline of osteopathy was founded by Andrew Taylor Still (1828–1917), an American physician who served as a surgeon during the Civil War. Frustrated by illogical therapies employed by organized medicine at the time, Dr. Still hypothesized that an integrated and balanced musculoskeletal structure was optimal for physiological functioning. Further, the body's structural function depended upon psychological, emotional, familial, and societal influences. The 26 osteopathic medical schools in the United States train doctors almost the same way as medical schools that award an M.D. (medical doctor) degree as opposed to a D.O. (doctor of osteopathic) degree. Most of the 78,000 osteopaths practice in a primary care, family practice, or internal medicine setting. However, their training also includes instruction in physical modalities such as myofascial release, cranial manipulation, and high-velocity, low-amplitude "thrusts," which benefit many of our fibromyalgia patients. Over the years, some of these techniques have found their way into general use by rehabilitation medicine physicians, physical therapists, and chiropractors.

How Do Chiropractors Manage Fibromyalgia?

In 1895, an Iowa healer named D. D. Palmer developed the theory that proper alignment of the spinal column allows unimpeded nerve flow to the soft tissues. This flow is necessary to achieve optimal health. If structural bones and body muscles are in proper alignment, the body should take over and heal itself. Unlike osteopaths, chiropractors do not practice internal medicine, perform surgery, or write prescriptions. In an effort to treat spinal *subluxations* (less than full dislocations) they use manual adjustments, manipulations, and "cracking" to force movements of body parts to increase range of motion and relax muscles There are 52,000 chiropractors in the United States, and 10% of the population visits them at least occasionally. Over the years, chiropractors have incorporated principles of rehabilitation medicine, physical therapy, occupational therapy, and osteopathy into their practice. We have found that their interventions generally are modestly beneficial to our fibromyalgia patients. Patients who seek chiropractic therapy should coordinate the modalities employed with their primary care physician, rheumatologist, physiatrist, or orthopedist. Controlled trials of chiropractic in fibromyalgia show modest results at best. There are many ways health care professionals can work together to improve their patients' health. Occasionally, some chiropractic approaches aggravate fibromyalgia-related pain. If this is the case, therapy should either be discontinued or discussed with the physician and chiropractor.

Investigational or Questionable Complementary Approaches

Naturopathy is based on the belief that disease can be treated by a return to nature in regulating the diet, deep-breathing exercises, bathing, and the employment of various forces to eliminate poisonous products from the system. While there is nothing wrong with using the healing powers of nature, in our opinion laxatives, purges that induce vomiting, and colonics are of no benefit for fibromyalgia and are potentially dangerous. *Naprapathy* deals with therapeutic manipulations and *Reiki* manipulates energy flow around the body without touching it. *Ayurveda* uses yoga and dietary modifications that present no problems, but also preaches that correct spiritual and physical balancing requires purification. These purifications include enemas, vomiting, and blood letting, which only aggravate fibromyalgia. *Reflexology* treats the ears, hands, and feet with manual stimulation as a way of treating the whole body. Based on the theory that specific areas of the ears, hands, and feet correspond to organs, glands, and nerves, reflexology makes no scientific sense but may help patients through a placebo effect in giving them time, attention, relaxation, pleasing sensations, and a sympathetic ear. As noted earlier in this chapter, many forms of *massage* clearly benefit patients. However, specific massage techniques such as rolfing and Hellerwork are too vigorous for most fibromyalgia patients and frequently induce more pain. These techniques may be appropriate for patients without fibromyalgia. Finally, the belief that *magnetic fields* influence energy and blood flow has had a resurgence of popularity since the introduction of MRI imaging as a diagnostic procedure. Some advocates of the *polarity theory* believe that magnets can balance energy forces of the body and apply magnets to various areas of the body. None of our patients who have done this have had any response to this treatment, for which there is little scientific basis.

SUMMING UP

A minority of fibromyalgia patients require a formalized rehabilitation program. When prescribed, it generally consists of a gradual exercise program, as well as physical and occupational therapy. Some form of counseling may be part of this program. The principal goals of any rehabilitation process should include reducing stress, promoting greater stamina and endurance, improving clarity of thought, avoiding discomfort at work and at home, showing patients how to carry on an independent exercise program, lessening reliance on medication, and improving the ability to cope with pain.

FOR FURTHER READING

Arthritis Foundation. *Your Personal Guide to Living Well with Fibromyalgia.* Atlanta, Georgia: Longstreet Press, 1997.

Jones KD, Adams D, Winters-Stone K, Burckhardt CS. A comprehensive review of 46 exercise treatment studies in fibromyalgia (1988–2005). *Health & Quality of Life Outcome*; 2006: *4*: 67.

Leventhal LJ. Management of fibromyalgia. *Annals Intern Med 131*, 1999: 850–858.

Martin DP, Sletten CD, Williams BA, Berger IH. Improvement in fibromyalgia symptoms with acupuncture: results of a randomized controlled trial. *Mayo Clin Proc* 2006; *81*: 749–757.

Sim J, Adams N. Systemic review of randomized controlled trials of nonpharmacological interventions for fibromyalgia. *Clinical J Pain* 2002; *18*: 324–336.

20
How to Overcome Fibromyalgia

All living souls welcome whatever they are ready to cope with; all else they ignore, or pronounce to be monstrous and wrong, or deny to be possible.
George Santayana (1863–1952),
Dialogues in Limbo, 1925

When our patients are diagnosed with fibromyalgia, their initial reaction generally is "What?" At this point, we provide them with literature from fibromyalgia support organizations and the Arthritis Foundation and explain what this condition means. Often we meet with family members to reinforce the educational process. In mild cases, this creates a sense of relief. Some patients who have seen several physicians and been given various diagnoses have differing reactions: "Are you just trying to put me off?" "My last rheumatologist said the same thing, told me he could do nothing for it, and sent me back to my family doctor." "Are you sure it's not lupus or Lyme disease or cancer?"

Once our patients have accepted the diagnosis and read about the syndrome, we examine their behavior patterns and try to find ways to help them deal with the diagnosis in a constructive manner. This chapter reviews some of the emotional reactions our patients display and problems they have to deal with, gives practical advice on how to surmount obstacles, and describes community resources that help patients overcome the syndrome.

THE PROBLEM: WHY COPING IS DIFFICULT

It's hard enough to get through the day when feeling unwell. In fibromyalgia, the sense of being unwell is manifested by fatigue, pain, spasm, poor sleeping, lack of stamina or endurance, and sometimes difficulty concentrating or focusing. Fibromyalgia patients frequently react to these sensations with specific attitudes, emotions, and other behavioral responses, including anxiety, anger, guilt, loss of self-esteem, depression, and fear.

You Look Great! How Could You Be Sick?

There are no physical markers of fibromyalgia that reveal the syndrome to others. Fibromyalgia patients have no deformities, don't have an *X* marked on their forehead, look healthy, and seem able to be active. While this is good for the patient in one sense, friends, employers, and loved ones often have difficulty believing that they have so many complaints. Therefore, it's important to be open and frank with those who care. You need to have their trust to help them understand the limitations imposed by fibromyalgia. Patients do not need to be coddled or treated like invalids; they crave and need understanding and respect. Tell those who care that with a few modifications and a little time, you can still be as productive and as much fun to be with as before.

Anxiety

Anxiety is fear of one's self

Wilhelm Stekel (1868–1940)

Anxiety is present in up to 70% of patients with fibromyalgia at some point during the course of the syndrome. It can be manifested by shortness of breath, palpitations, dizziness, lightheadedness, sweaty palms, trembling, chest pains, nausea, hot flashes, and, in extreme cases, a sense of impending doom or panic. Anxiety, in turn, worsens fibromyalgia symptoms, which sometimes can be hard to differentiate from those of anxiety. Anxiety is distressing but, if confronted firmly, will pass. Examine the causes of anxiety, face them, and don't run away. Patients must learn to relax and master their minds and bodies. Practice deep breathing, try to create a comfortable environment, write, or listen to pleasant music. Find ways to get a sense of control, dissipate the tensions of the day, create a sense of well-being, and get a good night's sleep.

Loss of Self-Esteem

Be a friend to thyself and others will be so too.

Thomas Fuller, M.D. (1654–1734),
Gnomologia, 1732

Fibromyalgia is a formidable syndrome that can lead to loss of self-esteem. Hurting and being tired all the time takes its toll. Some patients cannot meet educational or career goals, lose the ability to be self-supporting, cannot engage community activities, or experience cognitive impairment and difficulty focusing. This may lead to unstable or failed relationships with family and friends with consequent loss of self-esteem.

The first thing a fibromyalgia patient needs to be aware of is a self-esteem problem. How did this happen? What can be done about it? Several steps can improve self-esteem in a fibromyalgia patient. Achieving a sense of personal worth promotes self-confidence. Visualize being happy. Do things that are enjoyable or help others. Stop being negative. Develop affirmations. I am courageous, I have options; I am not a victim; I am learning to relax; I can solve it. Peer counseling is frequently helpful in this situation. Getting back one's self-esteem is one of the first steps toward overcoming fibromyalgia.

Anger

It's my rule never to lose my temper until it would be detrimental to keep it.
Sean O'Casey (1884–1964),
The Plough and the Stars, 1926

Patients who get upset because they are not feeling well aggravate their fibromyalgia by tightening their muscles, making relaxation impossible. There are several self-help steps to confronting anger. First, conduct a personal reality check. Is there anything actually wrong with the way things are going? Are your loved ones healthy and alive? How are things financially? Don't get upset over things beyond your control, such as traffic jams or long lines at the supermarket. Deal with life's stresses in nonconfrontational ways. When making phone calls that require being on hold for a while, watch television or listen to music while waiting. Don't run errands that might require standing in long lines if time is a problem. Don't blame people for causing your problems or illness. Anger can be energizing, but channel it positively. There are healthy ways to express bottled-up anger. Think of how to prevent getting angry and how to relieve anger when it builds. Keep a chart or diary to award accomplishments in dealing with problems. It will help create a sense of well being.

Guilt and Shame

Guilt, once harbored in the conscious breast, intimidates the brave, degrades the great.
Samuel Johnson (1709–1784)

Guilt has no place in fibromyalgia and makes the syndrome worse. Try to recognize its destructive effects. Regretting past behavior or thinking that you are bad are attitudes to be avoided. Don't berate yourself for things that fibromyalgia does not allow you to do. Overly perfectionistic tendencies can lead to guilt, as can unrealistic goal setting. Don't agonize over decisions that may have had unintended outcomes. We are all human, and we all make mistakes. Propose a rational response for dealing with guilt and looking ahead. Guilt is self-defeating. Develop a positive attitude to modify thoughts and behavior.

Depression

You handle depression in much the same way you handle a tiger....If depression is creeping up and must be faced, learn something about the nature of the beast: you may escape without a mauling.

R.W. Shepherd

In Chapter 17, we reviewed evidence that patients do not develop fibromyalgia because they are depressed, but that they can be depressed because they do not feel well. This reactive depression manifests as loss of interest and pleasure in life's daily activities. Classically defined as "helplessness and hopelessness," depression leads to a feeling of worthlessness, loss of appetite (or occasionally, overeating), altered sleep patterns, loss of self-esteem, inability to concentrate, guilt, complaints of fatigue, and loss of energy. Patients who are depressed have lower pain thresholds, lose interest in personal care and grooming, have trouble making decisions, and sometimes get into more accidents or arguments. Depression affects the body, moods, relationships, and physical activities.

In order to overcome depression, fibromyalgia patients must first recognize that it's a problem and express a desire to do something about it. Once an ounce of motivation is kindled, some of the techniques discussed in chapter 19 and later on in this chapter can be used to fight off depression. Medications prescribed to manage depression are reviewed in the next two chapters.

Perfectionism

Striving to better oft we mar what's well.

William Shakespeare (1564–1616),
King Lear, Act 1, sc. 4, 1. 369

Many of our fibromyalgia patients are overachievers. Prior to becoming ill, they led very busy lives with personal, work, and social commitments. A perfectionistic tendency is evident where every detail of each daily activity is comprehensively thought out and analyzed. This needs to be differentiated from a psychiatric disorder known as obsessive-compulsive behavior, which is reviewed in Chapter 17 and is not associated with fibromyalgia. When the symptoms of fibromyalgia manifest themselves, fatigue makes it difficult to accomplish all the patient used to be able to do, which in turn creates feelings of guilt and inadequacy when the patient cannot perform. This leads to fears of failure and rejection and difficulty handling criticism. Overachievers need to adjust, think innovatively, learn to budget their energy, and delegate responsibility. Don't get so bogged down in detail that the overall picture is lost. Let initial frustrations evolve into relaxation. Life is too precious to waste on details beyond our control!

Catastrophizing: Fear and trauma

The only thing we have to fear is fear itself—nameless unreasoning, unjustified terror which paralyzes needed efforts to convert retreat into advance.
                                        Franklin D. Roosevelt (1882–1945),
                                                    Inaugural Address, 1933

A minority of patients with fibromyalgia had something terrible happen to them in the past, which makes it harder to overcome pain, poor sleeping patterns, and spasm. They have a negative or pessimistic appraisal of their pain. They may have been a victim of abuse, neglect, a natural disaster, war, poverty, or a crime. Don't let others convince these patients that a single factor such as a virus, a specific diet, or a genetic tendency is solely responsible for the illness. Counseling is absolutely critical. Patients need to verbalize their traumas and the fears that go with them. They need to confront the facts of the situation and work out a way to get the past behind them so that their lives can go forward. This may require relocating to a safer environment, ending abusive relationships, or altering work styles. Only at this point can fibromyalgia be effectively overcome.

SOLUTIONS: HOW TO IMPROVE COPING SKILLS

As we have demonstrated, anxiety, fear, guilt, depression, loss of self-esteem, and anger are common emotions found in fibromyalgia patients. How should patients deal with these emotions and learn to cope better? Adequate coping requires taking action. Fasten your seat belts. We are going to do just that!

Develop Positive Goals and Attitudes

Holly was gorgeous and the envy of her friends. She always seemed in control and worked 18 hours a day building her communications consulting business. No detail was too small to be overlooked. But over several months, the fragile shell that nobody knew she had started to crack. After what seemed to be a mild flu, she began sleeping poorly and complaining of muscle spasms. Of course, Holly kept this to herself. However, when she started forgetting telephone numbers and a splitting headache nearly caused her to miss an important meeting, Holly consulted Dr. Gray. The work-up showed that Holly had fibromyalgia. Her perfectionistic tendencies enabled Holly to block the problem she was having forming serious relationships. Holly was lonely, and her family was 2,000 miles away.

Her immediate reaction was anger, which gave way to chronic anxiety. Although she reduced her workload, this only created a feeling of guilt. Dr. Gray referred her to a psychologist, who explained to Holly that her pain amplification was real and probably virally induced, but that unless she faced up to things in a positive, constructive manner, improvement would be much slower. Holly learned to manage her time and think positively. She learned how to relax and channel her frustration into energizing activities. Holly allowed herself time to go out on dates and rediscovered her sense of humor. She no longer takes fibromyalgia medication.

Patients should treat the diagnosis of fibromyalgia as a challenge to their resourcefulness. Like Holly, they should set realistic goals and be proactive. List all the problems, from easiest to hardest to resolve. Write down the remedies for each symptom, sign, and problem, one at a time. Follow the results. Reprioritize goals. Try not to do annoying, recurrent tasks. Don't be drawn into a no-win situation. Set limits and learn to say no. Avoid negative people. Instead of thinking that "It's hopeless and will never get better" or "This treatment will make me worse," try developing the attitude that things will get better and medication will help. Discuss medications with a doctor and inquire how they assist self-improvement. Decide if individual or group counseling is something that might expedite more positive feelings.

It's important to do positive things by challenging one's financial, personal, and intellectual resources. Cultivate spirituality. Develop new interests and hobbies. Seek positive news and information. Improve communication skills. If you are courteous and say "please" and "thank you," others will be helpful and pleasant in return. Give affection to others, and it will be returned. Don't worry about tomorrow; focus on what can be done today. Be open to receiving help and verbalizing thoughts; don't keep them suppressed. Patients who set attitude changes as goals really do start to feel better about themselves.

How to Improve Coping

Laurel always had low self-esteem. She worked installing turbines on an assembly line for a small, family-owned technology company. After several weeks, the pressure of carrying 50-pound boxes to the assembly area got to her. Laurel complained of pain in her back and shoulders and tingling in her hands. Over the next few months she found it increasingly difficult to sleep, and her abdomen became so distended that a friend asked her if she was pregnant. Laurel quit work after five months, but the pain did not go away. Dr. Lane noted that Laurel also reported headaches, palpitations, fatigue, low back discomfort, and stools filled with mucus. A diagnosis of fibromyalgia with irritable bowel syndrome was made. Her inability to hold the job made Laurel depressed and destroyed her self-confidence.

She seemed to be teary-eyed most of the time and was motivated to do nothing other than watch television and eat potato chips. Dr. Lane prescribed half a tablet of cyclobenzaprine (Flexeril) two hours before sleeping and Levsin for her bowel discomfort, and a week later added duloxetine (Cymbalta) in the morning. Since Laurel had lost her health insurance and could not afford counseling, Dr. Lane referred her to a local fibromyalgia support group, and Laurel took the Arthritis Foundation's "Fibromyalgia Self-Help Course." The course showed Laurel how to develop self-confidence and a positive outlook. Several months later, Laurel got a clerking job through a friend she met at the course and has held it for the past year. Dr. Lane intends to taper her medications soon.

In order to cope with fibromyalgia, be flexible and learn to adapt to the illness. Life can be happy in spite of fibromyalgia. Learn to understand the concept of self-responsibility and accept it. Most patients work, despite feeling unwell, by accommodating the illness. Explain what fibromyalgia is to spouses, relatives, and friends. The importance of seeking help and avoiding isolation cannot be overemphasized.

Dealing with Stress

Fern was getting it from all sides. Her mother had recently died, her son's business had gone bankrupt, and a flood caused severe damage to the home she had lived in for 30 years. Fern's stable fibromyalgia flared, and her lower back and neck pain was excruciating. Determined to overcome these obstacles, Fern took stock of herself. Her children were healthy, the house was insured, and she was happily married. She took alprazolam (Xanax) for three nights to alleviate the anxiety that had prevented her from sleeping. Fern rejoined her exercise class, which included deep-breathing exercises, stretching, and non-impact aerobics. Every morning, she performed isometric exercises for ten minutes. Whenever her husband noticed early signs of an inappropriate stress response, he made a point of warning her that she was getting anxious. Fern responded by practicing a biofeedback maneuver she had learned. She stopped volunteer work at an agency where her efforts were not appreciated and the work was too time-consuming. She made sure that there was time for herself during the day. Fern's fibromyalgia started to ease up.

In Chapters 3 and 6, we reviewed how stress or trauma can bring on fibromyalgia and reviewed the biochemical pathways by which this occurs. A recent survey suggested that 63% of fibromyalgia patients feel that stress is a major factor in influencing their symptoms, signs, and disease course.

How can stress be decreased? First, remember that lessening stress increases energy. In the beginning, learn to relax. Find a quiet environment and a comfortable position. Whether it's listening to soft music, practicing meditation, guided imagery, deep abdominal breathing, hypnosis, thinking of or inhaling pleasant aromas (*aromatherapy*), tai chi, prayer, or biofeedback, we support whatever works. Next, learn to say no and communicate your concerns. It may be necessary to accept limitations and modify job descriptions and workstations to limit physical and emotional stress. Budget time to allow for periods of relaxation. Learn to pace. Make a list of everything that is stressful and how these factors can be avoided or improved. Also, enjoy distractions. Have fun. Learn to laugh. Listen to comedy shows or tapes, read a good book, or take up gardening. Get a pet. Develop a hobby. Distractions make it easier to perform necessary or required activities that are less enjoyable. Finally, remember that stress can cause and aggravate fibromyalgia by releasing chemicals that aggravate or accelerate symptoms of pain and fatigue.

Develop a Positive Doctor-Patient Relationship

Never go to a doctor whose office plants have died.
                                                        Erma Bombeck (1927–1996)

Whether they are seeing a mental health therapist, physical therapist, chiropractor, or physician, patients must be able to communicate with their health care professionals. Since only physicians can prescribe medication or hospitalize, their relationships with and feelings toward patients are extremely important. Here are a few tips on how to maximize the doctor-patient relationship.

Find a doctor who believes that fibromyalgia exists and is interested in helping these patients. Avoid unreasonable expectations. Does the doctor have a genuine interest in the patient as a person? Does the physician reinforce the patient's self-esteem, listen, or allow disagreements or questions? Does the patient feel comfortable asking questions or feel too rushed? Does the doctor talk in plain English? Most important, will the doctor be the patient's advocate? Can he or she write jury duty letters, allow handicap placards if needed, fill out disability forms, and defend the patient in a legal deposition?

In return for these considerations, be sensitive to the doctor's needs. Be organized and honest. If it's hard to explain a problem, write it down and restrict the note to one page. What makes the complaint better or worse? What's been tried in the past? Do not argue with the doctor. Be informative and reasonable. Don't expect an instant cure. Follow the suggested course of therapy to completion—a noncompliant patient cannot expect to improve fully. Doctor-patient relationships are important partnerships that can be quite fragile at times. *Adherence* to medication and treatment recommendations are very important. Studies have shown only a 50% compliance rate with a rheumatologist's treatment plan.

If a physician referral is needed, call the nearest medical school, county medical association, Arthritis Foundation, or fibromyalgia support group.

HOW TO MOBILIZE RESOURCES

There are many people who really care about a fibromyalgia patient's health and well-being. Whether it be a spouse, family member, friend, or someone in the community, there are many resources that can be called upon in the treatment process. In the following sections, we describe the kinds of help that support people and groups can provide.

Marriage, Sexuality, and Family

Pains do not hold a marriage together. It is threads, hundreds of tiny threads which sew people together through the years... That's what makes a marriage last—more than passion or even sex.

Simone Signoret (1921–1985)

Marge had been married to Henry for five years when she sustained a whiplash injury in a motor vehicle accident. Though she did all the right things, her localized neck sprain evolved into full-blown fibromyalgia over several months. Marge complained of fatigue, aching, and irritable colon. She became sensitive to weather changes and had difficulty sleeping. Since she looked the same, Henry could not understand why Marge would not play golf with him on weekends or why she kept him up at night tossing and turning while trying to find a comfortable position. Henry's anger made things worse, and this affected their relationship. A classmate of Marge's sister at the university had fibromyalgia. The classmate's advice to the sister allowed Marge to confide her concerns to her parents and siblings. Marge rented a video on fibromyalgia from the Arthritis Foundation for Henry since he did not like to read. She took Henry to her next rheumatology visit, and Dr. March explained how Henry could be more understanding and supportive. Henry demonstrated greater insight, which indirectly helped Marge's fibromyalgia to improve.

Married or unmarried couples may wish to probe how their relationship interacts with fibromyalgia and vice versa. Make sure that the partner knows what fibromyalgia is and how he or she can help the patient enjoy life. Open communication decreases resentment and resolves potential conflict. Be on the lookout for potential problems. Does the partner resent or attempt to control the fibromyalgia patient? Does he or she buffer upsetting information before telling the patient? Does the mate derive satisfaction from caring for a fibromyalgia patient? Does the mate feel neglected or unable to help?

A good sexual relationship is a source of pleasure, self-esteem, and relaxation, which also decreases stress. Fibromyalgia should not interfere physiologically with lovemaking. The uncommon exceptions include autonomically mediated dry vaginal walls (easily treated with lubricants) and significant spasm of vaginal muscles, often with a history of sexual or physical abuse (see Chapter 13). Occasionally, fibromyalgia medications can influence libido. Don't be afraid to ask a doctor about the potential side effects of medications before taking them. Enhancing intimacy while reducing stress should be a goal.

Relatives and friends should be helpful resources. Some fibromyalgia patients react to the disease by decreasing their social contacts and isolating themselves. "I'm too tired to do anything" or "I hurt too much to be away for more than a few hours" are warning signs of a developing problem. When patients complain of difficulty keeping up with household chores or meeting responsibilities to their children, relationships may become precarious. The sleep disorder of fibromyalgia can also alter intimacy. Develop a positive plan to be an active family member, taking limitations into account. Keep all communication channels open with family members. They should be a patient's biggest cheerleaders!

Sometimes, family strife can worsen fibromyalgia. If this is the case, identify the sources of stress that interfere with rehabilitation. Focus on the problems, develop means for dealing with them positively, and seek counseling if needed.

Community Resources and Self-help Groups

Therefore the moon, the governess of floods, Pale in her anger; washes all the air, That rheumatic diseases do abound.
William Shakespeare (1564–1616),
A Midsummer Night's Dream, Act 2, Sc. 34, 1. 105

Appendix 1 lists agencies and organizations that assist fibromyalgia patients. A self-help group usually consists of 5–20 members who meet on a regular basis (usually once a month) to share information and experiences. The group leader should allow time for questions and answers, give research and clinical updates, and permit presentations by health care professionals. The leader should be strong yet empathetic, not allow one person to dominate the sessions, and set a positive, constructive tone. Members develop friendships that often provide additional support systems.

Finally, we need to address the Internet. Fibromyalgia patients surfing the Internet will find three basic sources of information: legitimate research and summaries of clinical papers put together by fibromyalgia support organizations or medical society websites; entrepreneurs trying to sell dietary or medically unproven remedies; and chat rooms where information, personal experiences, and concerns are shared. Try to stick to the sites recommended by the Arthritis Foundation or fibromyalgia support organizations. Don't try any unproven therapeutic approach unless you discuss it with a doctor.

CIRCUMSTANCES THAT WARRANT SPECIAL CONSIDERATION

When fibromyalgia attacks a child or an older individual or is present during pregnancy, consider the advice provided in the following sections.

Dealing with Fibromyalgia in Children and Adolescents

Phillip was ten when he complained of pain in his legs. The pediatrician thought it was growing pains and reassured Phillip's mother. When it persisted, X-rays of the painful areas and blood tests were done—both were normal. Ultimately, Phillip was referred to a pediatric rheumatologist, who found tender points in his knees, upper back and neck, and buttock regions. Dr. Park diagnosed Phillip as having juvenile fibromyalgia. He was started on ibuprofen. Phillip's mother went to the school and arranged for him to have a ground-level locker, made sure that his teachers noticed when his knapsack was too heavy, and checked that Phillip always attached the pack to his back. She also met with Coach Adams and showed him the types of exercises the rheumatologist recommended and the ones Phillip should avoid. Phillip was concerned that his friends would single him out for ridicule in view of his special needs, but the sixth-grade teachers handled the situation so deftly that none of his classmates really noticed.

As reviewed in Chapter 16, fibromyalgia is extremely uncommon in children. As a result, they often feel alone. Ask them to explain their pain. Make sure it's not a growing pain or early juvenile rheumatoid arthritis. Is reflex sympathetic dystrophy part of the syndrome? If so, this mandates a comprehensive rehabilitation program.

At school, don't let teachers accuse the child of being lazy. Educate them about the syndrome. Make things easier for the child, but assign them chores. Have the child use a knapsack that balances weight properly. Allow and encourage the use of markers or felt-tipped pens, which make writing easier. Don't stigmatize the child. Talk to the physical education instructor. Use colorful splints if needed. Ask the child what he or she thinks will be helpful at school and at home. Children are often afraid to verbalize their concerns.

Adolescents with fibromyalgia may be noncompliant in taking medications that alter mood, behavior, or appearance. All too often, doctors are unaware of this. Teenage girls often mistake menstrual symptoms for those of fibromyalgia. Adolescents need a role model apart from the immediate family to help them through difficult times. Whether the teen turns to a relative, coach, teacher, or clergyman, encourage this type of interaction. Talk to school officials and teachers. Encourage participation in extracurricular activities that don't aggravate fibromyalgia and allow the development of self-esteem and self-respect.

Wrestling is out, but the school newspaper or yearbook, certain exercise classes, French club, or drama club are possible.

Fibromyalgia and Pregnancy

Ellen had mild fibromyalgia controlled with intermittent pregabalin (Lyrica) when she learned that her first child was on its way. After consulting the *Physicians Desk Reference (PDR)* in a bookstore, she stopped taking Lyrica. After several weeks, Ellen was in agony; her muscles and joints were stiff and achy. Dr. Rose told her to take acetaminophen (Tylenol) for the aches and acquainted her with literature suggesting that Elavil was safe during pregnancy. After she delivered a healthy daughter, Ellen's fibromyalgia flared again as a result of nightly feedings that deprived her of sleep. Every time she carried her daughter, Ellen winced in pain. She had stopped taking Elavil so that she could breast-feed, but Dr. Rose made her aware of literature showing that the immunologic protective advantages of breast-feeding do not extend beyond the first three months of life. Ellen occasionally took Tylenol for three months and weaned the baby so that she could go back on Lyrica when necessary. Her husband was now able to help with the feedings, and Dr. Rose showed Ellen how to carry the baby so that minimal stress was put on her upper back muscles.

To our surprise, every year a patient of ours undergoes a therapeutic abortion because she believes that pregnancy has made her fibromyalgia too painful or that she will not be able to care for the baby. Women with fibromyalgia have fewer pregnancies than individuals without the syndrome. Some patients have told me that it would be impossible to get by without their medication and that they worry about its effects on the unborn.

What really happens during pregnancy? Pregnancy can aggravate fibromyalgia, but this happens only 20–30% of the time. Problems are associated more with sleep deprivation, hormonal changes, breast enlargement producing myofascial discomfort, morning stiffness, leg cramps, and low back pain, especially during the last trimester. Fatigue also can be a major problem. Yet, most of our patients do rather well and view these problems as worthwhile inconveniences considering the fulfillment of having a child. Even though manufacturers cannot guarantee successful pregnancies if their drugs are used, and routinely place warnings in the *PDR,* studies suggest that pregnant women can take acetaminophen (Tylenol) and some FM medications in their usual dose without worrying. Patients should consult with their doctor to ascertain wheat is safe in your circumstance.

Sometimes fibromyalgia flares after delivery, especially if it is associated with postpartum depression. If medication is needed, be prepared to stop breast-feeding early or do not breast-feed at all. This gives the doctor greater flexibility in recommending medication. Carry the baby in a way that straddles the weight so as not to produce too much myofascial tension. Have the spouse handle some nighttime feedings to minimize sleep disruption. If financially feasible, consider hiring someone to help with baby care and housework. Many communities have mommy's helpers programs through churches or community centers. The temporary inconveniences caused by pregnancy should be viewed as minor nuisances on a road that ultimately yields tremendous dividends!

Fibromyalgia in the Elderly

As time passed, people saw less of Frances. She started to miss bridge games and thought of excuses not to have lunch with her friends. Frances told them she was too tired and achy, the weather was bad, or she had a doctor's appointment. Her fibromyalgia medication was no longer being taken regularly, and Frances showed less enjoyment of life and decreased interest in interacting with friends. Frances's daughter accompanied her on her next doctor's visit and explained her concerns to Dr. Frank. He put Frances on nortriptyline (Pamelor), a tricyclic, in a dose also used to treat depression. Frances's daughter made sure that her mother would no longer be able to isolate herself. Within weeks she hurt less and slept better, and her old personality started to come back.

Fibromyalgia rarely develops in older patients for the first time, but as patients with the syndrome age, their problems grow. In addition to all the considerations previously noted in this chapter, there are a few additional points that warrant discussion.

First, some of the concerns we expressed about social isolation, communication skills, and community interactions need to be emphasized in elderly people. Once older persons cut themselves off from social outlets and stay indoors, their fibromyalgia worsens and their ability to function independently is impaired. Make sure that your senior-citizen friend, colleague, or relative remains a viable member of the community. Also, doctors tend to put elderly patients on more medication. Whether they help the heart, blood pressure, lung, prostate, or diabetes, many of these agents interfere with fibromyalgia preparations. Some can worsen sexual performance; others can cause depression, promote aching or fatigue, or interfere with the ability to get around by producing lightheadedness or dizziness. Ask a doctor how any newly prescribed drug will influence fibromyalgia or interact with other medications given for particular health problems.

Older individuals need less sleep but are more affected by sleep medications, which produce dizziness or mental clouding. The development of osteoarthritis and osteoporosis with age tends to blur the distinction between fibromyalgia and another musculoskeletal diagnosis. Work with the family, community, and doctor to make the golden years truly golden.

SUMMING UP

Fibromyalgia patients frequently express feelings of anger, guilt, anxiety, and depression, which also aggravate the disease. There are ways to channel these feelings constructively, improve coping, relieve stress, devise positive goals, and assume favorable attitudes to make things better. Develop strategies, priorities, and organization, along with a support system of family, friends, co-workers, and the community, to stand up to the challenge of fibromyalgia.

FOR FURTHER READING

Koulil SV, Effting M, Kraaimaat FW, van Lankveld W, van Helmand T, Cats H, van Riel PLCM. Cognitive-behavioral therapies and exercise programmes for patients with fibromyalgia: State of the art and future directions. *Ann Rheum Dis* 2007; *66*: 571–581.

Wallace DJ, Clauw DJ, Hallegua DS. Addressing behavioral abnormalities in fibromyalgia. *J Musculoskeletal Medicine* 2005; *22*: 562–579.

21

Evaluating Medicines That Work for Fibromyalgia

The best practitioners give to their patients the least medicine.
Frederick Saunders (1807–1902)

Nobody likes to take medicine. Many fibromyalgia patients, in particular, prefer to treat their condition with natural remedies, and many are reluctant to take prescribed medication. This problem is made more difficult because many of the most helpful preparations are designated as antidepressants. Some patients become concerned that this might create a stigma. "If you really believe what I am saying, and are convinced that I am not crazy, why are you giving me an anti-depressant or antianxiety drug?" is a question we frequently hear. This problem is compounded when some insurance companies refuse to reimburse patients for these preparations, claiming that they are uncovered "psychiatric benefits."

Management of fibromyalgia includes medications from separate families or groups, in which we list at least one agent that has been shown in double-blinded, controlled trials (where some of the study subjects get placebo, or sugar pills) to be effective in fibromyalgia patients. The rationale for using these drugs in treating fibromyalgia is reviewed in this chapter, but first the scientific logic behind putting these drugs on our "A" list will be discussed.

THE BURDEN OF PROOF

How Is a Drug Shown to Be Effective in Managing a Disorder?

In the United States, the Food and Drug Administration (FDA) approves drugs for specific indications. It takes many years and many dollars for an agent to be approved for a specific use, and since fibromyalgia was not recognized as a disorder until 1990, currently three have FDA approval for the condition.

Many of the remedies purported to help fibromyalgia are beyond the FDA's regulatory control. These include a variety of vitamins and agents that are licensed as food supplements. As a result, promising preparations such as DHEA and melatonin (reviewed in Chapter 22) are widely available without a prescription and are being taken by patients even though few controlled trials have documented their safety or efficacy. For example, there is no legal obligation to prove that a 3-mg tablet of melatonin really contains 3 mg. Also, each batch of medication can be mixed with varying preservatives, which may affect its delivery, or bioavailability. Some of our patients have no difficulty taking the medication but react to its packaging.

Physicians who manage fibromyalgia patients must rely on scientific studies showing that a drug is effective in alleviating a particular condition. These studies use different levels of proof. When a remedy is thought to be potentially helpful for a condition it was not designed or created for, a physician usually submits a *case report* to a medical journal. Journals recognized by a committee under the direction of the National Library of Medicine in Bethesda, Maryland, as having high *peer review* standards are listed in *Index Medicus* or *PubMed* and are also available for on-line referencing. These journals evaluate all materials submitted to them by physicians, allied health professionals, or basic science experts. Papers that meet a certain standard are considered for publication, usually after the editors make comments or constructive suggestions to improve the submission. The rigor of the review and the quality of material submitted to a publication are in turn interpreted by physicians who decide to subscribe to or read the journal or ask their local medical library to obtain it. For example, the *New England Journal of Medicine* accepts less than 10% of the manuscripts submitted to it for publication, whereas other journals' acceptance rate can be as high as 70%. Articles appearing in medical journals not recognized by the National Library of Medicine should create a healthy skepticism in the reader's mind. For instance, if the breakthrough being claimed was so dramatic, why wouldn't a peer-reviewed, recognized journal publish it?

If a compelling case report on the effectiveness of a specific treatment for a disorder is published, it is usually followed by case reports or a series of cases. In other words, practitioners like to see that an approach is helpful in more than one patient, hopefully in more than one institution or office setting. If a large number of patients feel better when taking a drug in an *open-label* fashion (where they know what they are receiving), investigators usually design a drug trial. The complexity of drug trials varies considerably; some of the options available to an investigator are as follows:

1. *Retrospective trial*—the experiences of all patients who took a drug previously in a particular setting are analyzed.
2. *Prospective trial*—a study is initiated before the drug's use is started and the drug is evaluated as time goes on.
3. *Controlled trial*—study patients are compared with a group of individuals not getting the drug. They can be matched by race, ethnicity, age, socioeconomic level, geography, or other variables.

4. *Blinded trial*—patients do not know what they are getting, but their doctors do. Patients are given a lot of personal attention in a drug trial and thus may feel better even though they are given a placebo; this must be factored into any study.
5. *Double blinded trial*—neither the patients nor the doctors know if the patients are getting the drug or a placebo.
6. *Multicenter trial*—the study is conducted in several locations.

The most convincing results are obtained when a double-blinded, international, multicenter, prospective, placebo-controlled trial using a large number of patients demonstrates a drug's ameliorative effects.

HOW DO WE MEASURE THE EFFECTIVENESS OF A DRUG FOR FIBROMYALGIA?

How Are Drugs Evaluated for Fibromyalgia?

The Food and Drug Administration evaluates drugs for potential use in a condition such as FM on the basis of clinical trials. Trials are conducted as Phase I, II, III, or IV initiatives. Usually drugs are given to animals before being tested in humans. Only 3% of the agents studied for all diseases ever make it to market.

Phase I studies are done to identify the proper dose ranges for which an investigational agent can be administered while monitoring and studying the method of absorption and possible toxicity of a new agent. Usually the first 20–100 subjects are healthy volunteers. Participants may be confined for 24-hour periods at special overnight research centers where they are closely studied and monitored with frequent questionnaires, and blood and urine tests.

Phase II studies evaluate the safety and effectiveness in 100–300 patients who have a targeted disease or condition. They take 1–3 years to complete and are geared towards adjusting treatment doses. Standard treatments or placebo are the usual comparitors. If results are favorable, sometimes an "open label" continuation of the study is available.

Phase III trials provide the facts about an investigational drug through extensive testing of the safety, efficacy, and proper dosage levels in a large group of patients. Usually, several thousand patients participate in these trials, which are often randomized, double-blind, prospective, placebo-controlled efforts.

Phase IV trials usually involve studying a drug that is already approved for a new indication and is often open label.

Many drugs already on the market have been suggested to be useful in FM and were studied outside of the FDA umbrella. *Levels of evidence* rate the quality of answering the primary research question for a therapeutic (does a drug work?), prognostic (outcome), or diagnostic (investigating a diagnostic test) study or developing an economic or decision model (is it cost effective?). These efforts are commonly rated as follows:

Level I is a high quality randomized trial with statistically significant differences.

Level II is a lesser quality randomized controlled trial (e.g., no blinding).

Level III is a case control study or retrospective comparative study.

Level IV is a case series.

Level V consists of expert opinion.

There are four grades of recommendation: A—supported by good evidence (Level 1 studies with consistent findings); B—supported by fair evidence (includes Level II and III studies); C—conflicting or poor quality evidence (Level IV or V studies) which do not allow for a recommendation for or against an intervention.

Fewer than 1% of all published FM publications in the last 40 years are Level I with a grade of A. Hence, interpreting the literature is often problematic.

METHODS OF CLINICAL ASCERTAINMENT AND ASSESSMENT

Fibromyalgia patients seen in a clinical practice setting have multiple symptoms, signs, laboratory findings and coexisting conditions. There is no single measure, metric, or index that allows a treating practitioner to assess in a reliable, efficient manner how a FM patient is responding to a therapeutic intervention. Simply listening to a patient after examining him or her is not sufficient. The Food and Drug Administration and the fibromyalgia subcommittee of OMERACT (Outcome Measures in Rheumatology) have analyzed the situation and come up with guidance recommendations that led to three agents being approved for the syndrome. The available inventories and methodologies are summarized in Table 21.1. A critical review of these is beyond the scope of this monograph, but all the domains numerically listed should be considered.

The most reliable indices are felt to be the FIQ, or Fibromyalgia Impact Questionnaire and the PGIC, or Patient and Global Impression of Change as well as the Mean Daily Average Pain ratings. The FIQ consists of a 20-item questionnaire that covers eight domains: physical functioning, days feeling well, work, pain, fatigue, morning stiffness, anxiety, and depression. The PGIC rates change on a scale of 11. A "minimally clinical important difference" is felt to be a 30% change.

Table 21.1. *Inventories and Methodologies Used in Fibromyalgia Studies and Clinical Trials*

1. Evaluating Pain
   Visual analog scale
   McGill Pain Questionnaire
   Tender point evaluations
   Leeds Assessment of Neuropathic Symptoms and Signs
   Brief Pain Inventory
   Dolorimetry
2. Patient and Global Impression of Change (PGIC)*
3. Fatigue
   Multidimensional Assessment of Fatigue
   Functional Assessment of Chronic Illness Therapy
   Fatigue Severity Scale
4. Sleep
   Medical Outcomes Sleep Scale
   Pittsburg Sleep Quality Index
   Jenkins Sleep Scale
5. Function and quality of life
   Fibromyalgia Impact Questionnaire *
   Short-Form-36 (SF-36) Health Survey
   Health Assessment Questionnaire
   Sexual functioning inventories
6. Psychological evaluations
   Beck Depression Inventory
   Beck Anxiety Inventory
   Mini International Neuropsychiatric Interview
   Hospital Anxiety and Depression Scale
   Hamilton Depression Rating Scale
   Stress-Trait Anxiety Inventory
   Coping Strategies Questionnaire
   Nottingham Health Profile Score
   Catastrophizing strategies
7. Tenderness
   Tender point count
   Pressure pain threshold measurement
8. Neurocognitive state (dyscognition)
9. Objective biomarkers
   Cytokine indices
   Quantitative brain imaging

* Used by the FDA to approve agents and found to be the most reliable by OMERACT and consensus documents.

SUMMING UP

Over a thousand remedies have been purported to improve fibromyalgia. Fewer than 1% have achieved a Level I evidence A grade in published studies. There is an urgent need for more high quality FM investigators to be trained and trials initiated. Literature reviews suggest that some approaches are more successful than others and are reviewed in the next chapter.

FOR FURTHER READING

Arnold LM, Williams DA, Hudson JI. *et al.* Development of responder definitions for fibromyalgia clinical trials. *Arthritis Rheum* 2012; *64*: 885–894.

Bennett R. The Fibromyalgia Impact Questionnaire (FIQ): A review of its development, current version, operating characteristics and uses. *Clinical Experimental Rheum* 2005; *23* (Supp 39): S154–S162.

Mease PJ. Assessment of patients with fibromyalgia syndrome. *J Musculoskeletal Pain* 2008; *16*: 75–80.

22

Drugs That May Be Useful in Fibromyalgia Patients: An Overview

Life as we find it is too hard for us; it entails too much pain, too many dis-appointments, impossible tasks. We cannot do without palliative remedies.
                                                    Sigmund Freud (1856–1939),
                                        Civilization and Its Discontents, 1930

This chapter will review both non-pharmacologic and pharmacologic approaches toward fibromyalgia that have been shown to have some efficacy in clinical studies and trials. In one survey of 30 studies conducted between 1980 and 2010, 3,846 patients received placebo therapy. The authors found that 31% had a 30% reduction of pain (the minimally clinical important difference), and 19% had a 50% reduction of pain. Clearly, putting patients in an environment where they are given "tender, loving care," attention, and concern may be as effective as giving medication. As noted in Chapter 21, the OMERACT consensus was that five components were important in evaluating clinical trials in FM: FIQ total score; reduction in pain (e.g., PGIC); 30% reduction in pain; improved sleep and sleep quality. Ernest Choy's group in Great Britain reported in 2011 that a search of all pertinent databases found 577 drug trials in fibromyalgia; 113 included duplicate publications, and only 21 used the OMERACT-recommended components. Therefore, a lot of what is reviewed in this section is based on consensus and experience, largely due to the poor quality of published studies in this area.

LOCALIZED REMEDIES

Most patients with myofascial pain syndrome can avoid long-term systemic therapies. Local approaches include injections and topical agents (Table 22.1). Their effectiveness has not been well studies in randomized clinical trials, and may be dependent upon regional variation in drug penetration, concentration gradients, dosing schedules, and vehicles (e.g., cream, ointment, lotion, occlusive dressing).

Do Tender Point Injections Work?

One of the most commonly employed interventions in fibromyalgia is the *tender point injection.* Controlled studies have clearly demonstrated its usefulness in patients with myofascial pain syndrome. When a patient comes to our office and reports that a specific point—for example, in the upper back or neck area—hurts, we try to ascertain how severe this discomfort is in relation to their overall pain. If we are told that at least 30% (and preferably more than 50%) of their pain at the moment is from a specific tender area, this is an indication for a local injection. Patients who "hurt all over" rarely respond to tender point injections for more than a few days.

Once we have decided to give a local injection or injections (usually limiting the number of injections to three per visit, with visits spaced several weeks apart), what preparations are used? The drugs of choice always include a local pain deadener, or anesthetic, usually Xylocaine, Novocaine, or Marcaine. After the painful area is sprayed with a coolant anesthetic such as ethyl chloride or florimethane, the anesthetic in the shots usually works immediately. Sometimes a steroid is added to the anesthetic in the same syringe.

Not all doctors use steroids for tender point injections. However, the doses we use are very low, and systemic effects are uncommon. The recommended preparations include triamcinolone (Kenalog or Aristocort), which is the most useful but must be given carefully since it sometimes dissolves fat tissue around the injection site and leaves a "pit"; betamethasone (Celestone), which is quite effective but burns more than other brands; methylprednisolone (Depo-Medrol), which does not last as long as the others but is well tolerated; and dexamethasone (Decadron LA), which is mild and well tolerated. The full benefits of these injections are usually apparent within several days, although patients may complain of local pain, flushing, or tingling for the first one or two days. The physician has to be very careful when injecting the upper back areas. He or she usually grasps or "lifts up" an area of fat or fascia to avoid puncturing the lung, a temporarily painful condition known as a *pneumothorax.* Pneumothorax is the most critical complication of the procedure, although it is very rare. Local injections can be given as often as needed, but we have found them worthwhile only if they provide relief for at least several weeks.

Figure 22.1 illustrates a tender point injection.

What about Botox Injections?

Botox is a form of botulinum toxin Type A, a bacterial-derived substance that relaxes muscles through inhibition of alpha motor neurons. Approved by the FDA for strabismus and blepharospasm (lazy eye and constant winking), in controlled studies Botox injections clearly help some headaches and decreases neck pain secondary to whiplash. Some investigators have noted that some patients

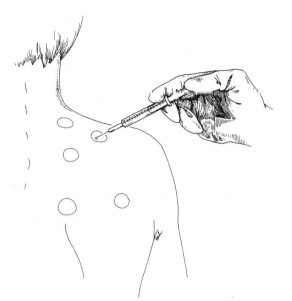

Fig. 22.1. *Example of a tender point injection.*

have had several months of relief after injecting it into tender points. Injections into the pelvic musculature have improved chronic pelvic pain. Botox should only be used by practitioners experienced with its administration and can be quite expensive.

Do Nerve Blocks or Epidurals work?

Nerve blocks are anesthetics and/or steroids injected into nerve tissues to relieve pain. Severe, localized, painful manifestations of reflex sympathetic dystrophy respond to nerve blocks, especially in the stellate ganglion area of the shoulder region.

Many patients with regional myofascial pain are incorrectly diagnosed as having herniated discs or arthritic disorders of the spine on the basis of abnormal X-rays, CT scans, or MRI scans. Unless an EMG with a nerve conduction study confirms that these abnormalities are producing physiologic changes, these X-ray or scanning results should be viewed with some skepticism. A study of healthy, asymptomatic people in their 40s who volunteered to have spinal MRI scans showed that 30% of them had significant abnormalities that rarely if ever caused symptoms. We have many fibromyalgia and myofascial pain syndrome patients who received epidural spinal nerve blocks for nonspecific radiographic abnormalities and localized symptoms that mimicked a disc disorder. The steroid in these epidural blocks often worsens the symptoms of fibromyalgia (see Chapter 13). Nerve blocks are usually recommended only if there is clear evidence of a herniated disc or a degenerative process called *spinal stenosis*.

When Are Local Salves Used?

Topical gels, creams, ointments, and lotions have been used to treat local pain. Believe it or not, agents containing *capsaicin* (Zostrix, Dolorac) are cayenne pepper derivatives that locally deplete substance P (a pain neurotransmitter). These preparations frequently burn but are otherwise harmless and take a week or so to work. Many other salves contain camphor or menthol which are soothing. Give yourself the rheumatologist's version of the "Pepsi challenge"! Apply capsaicin for one week to one side of the body and see if it feels better than the other side. Other local preparations include *topical NSAIDs and aspirin* (e.g., ketoprofen, diclofenac [Voltaren Gel], Aspercreme, Ben Gay) as well as neurotransmitter blockers (e.g., amitriptyline, cyclobenzaprine, gabapentin). Topical anesthesia in the form of *EMLA* (eutectic mixtures of local anasthetics), *Lidoderm* or *Tegaderm* block local pain for several hours by stabilizing nerve cell membranes.

Additional Topical, Physical Measures, and Devices

Some practitioners use topical traditional Chinese medicine. Physical therapists employ heat, ultrasound, phonopheresis (using ultrasound to drive pharmacologic agents such as corticosteroids, Xylocaine or Lidocaine subdermally into subcutaneous tissues), and transcutaneous electrical nerve stimulation. Balneotherapy involves bathing in mineral-containing waters, hot springs, or the use of mud baths, and this has been shown to be effective in randomized, controlled trials. However, most of these interventions have not been studied using adequate evidence-based methodologies, but are generally harmless and some patients report considerable benefits.

SYSTEMIC MEDICATIONS

Overview

In 2005, the Food and Drug Administration summarized the results of hearings and issued a guidance document to industry that established a roadmap for drugs to receive approval for a FM indication. As of this writing, three agents have been approved for fibromyalgia. A large 2012 survey found that nearly 2000 well-described FM patients were taking 182 different agents for FM. The most commonly used were duloxetine (26.8%); nonsteroidal anti-inflammatory drugs (26.6%); pregabalin (24.5%); opioids (24.2%); tramadol (15.3%); benzodiazepines (15.2%); cyclobenzaprine (12.9%); and milnacipran (8.9%). Most patients took at least two medications concurrently (77.8%). Only one-third, however, had a high level of continuous adherence to their regimen.

Agents Approved by the FDA for Fibromyalgia

Pregabalin (Lyrica) is a ligand for alpha-2-delta subtype 1 and 2 receptors that adhere to voltage-gated calcium channels and reduces calcium flux in neurons.

Table 22.1. *Topical Therapies Used by Fibromyalgia Patients*

Trigger point injections
Lidocaine or similar agents
Dry needling
Steroids
Botulinum toxin
Topical remedies
Salicylates
Nonsteroidals
Anticonvulsants (e.g., gabapentin)
Anesthetics (e.g., lidocaine)
Capsaicin
Antidepressants
Traditional Chinese medicines
Physical measures
Massage
Balneotherapy
Heat therapy
Ultrasound
Phonopheresis
Local electrical stimulation (e.g., TENS)

This reduces the release of substance P, glutamate, and norepinephrine, which results in analgesia and less anxiety. Using the mean pain score as the primary endpoint and patient global impression of change and the Fibromyalgia Impact Questionnaire as secondary endpoints, just about half of patients had a 30% response in doses of 300 mg to 600 mg daily. Its major side effects noted included dizziness, somnolence, weight gain, and edema, causing about 20% of volunteers to discontinue participation who were on real drug in the pivotal clinical trials. Many practitioners have found that some patients do well in doses as low as 75 mg daily. Patients often tolerate these compounds much better if most of the drug is given at bedtime. Pregabalin is also FDA approved for seizures and neuropathic pain (especially diabetic and post-shingles). We start with 75 mg at bedtime and build up from there with twice daily dosing.

Duloxetine (Cymbalta) is a serotonin-norepinephrine re-uptake inhibitor (SNRI) that has been on the market in the United States for generalized anxiety disorder, diabetic neuropathy, post herpetic neuralgia, and depression since 2005. In approximately 1,500 patients enrolled in four pivotal trials in FM, pain, global impression, fatigue, and function were shown to improve. The studies showed starting at 30 mg daily and working up to 60mg to 120mg a day was particularly effective. Duloxetine is also approved for chronic musculoskeletal pain associated with osteoarthritis. 19% of patients receiving drug discontinued their participation in the clinical trials due to adverse reactions.

Milnacipran (Savella) is another SNRI that has been available to manage depression in Europe and Japan for over 20 years, and this compound is approved for FM (but not depression) in the United States. This compound showed similar overall effects to duloxetine, with additional possible benefits in treating cognitive problems that are often seen in FM. These effects occurred at both 100 and 200mg per day. About one-third of patients who take milnacipran improve by about one-third. All SNRIs have a similar side effect profile, with nausea, constipation, postural dizziness, and palpitations as common adverse reactions leading 25% of milnacipran patients to stop the clinical trial. Milnacipran has no effect upon sleep. The nausea may be reduced by taking the drug with food, and the other side effects are often self-limited, and dissipate with time, and can be minimized by starting at a low dose and escalating slowly. Most practitioners start their patients on as little as 12.5 mg daily and build up to 50 to 100 mg twice daily.

Many practitioners combine pregabalin with duloxetine or milnacipran, and most use lower doses than reported in clinical trials. In our opinion, many other agents are much less costly and as effective as these three agents, but only the approved drugs have been studied in great detail.

Tricyclic Antidepressants

Tricyclic antidepressants (TCAs) have been available for more than 40 years and represent the old, reliable approach to managing fibromyalgia. In doses lower than those demonstrated to alleviate depression, TCAs have a variety of beneficial effects on the syndrome. First, they may increase the amount of delta wave sleep. Second, they improve the availability of serotonin to nerve cells. Third, they heighten the effect of endorphins, which decreases pain. Finally, they relax muscles. These actions are accomplished by the combined effect of increasing levels of serotonin, dopamine, and norepinephrine, acting as an antihistamine, as well as effects mediated via N-methyl d-aspartate antagonism and/or sodium channel blocking activity and decreasing parasympathetic autonomic activity. TCAs are not addictive, have no narcotic effect, and only indirectly decrease pain. These agents are inexpensive and available as generics.

In our experience, approximately one third of patients given a TCA report improvement in their FM symptoms. Their principal side effects include sicca (drying) symptoms, fatigue, and weight gain. A 2005 study critically reviewed 21 double-blind, placebo-controlled TCA trials published since 1986. The most commonly studied outcome measures included pain, visual assessment scales, physician global assessments, fatigue scales, dolorimetry, pain inventories, tender point examinations, tenderness measurements, and quality of life questionnaires. Four of the studies had a negative outcome; 17 demonstrated statistically significant responses using at least two of the metrics.

Which Tricyclic Should Be Used?

Sarah had mild fibromyalgia but tried to avoid taking medication because she was very sensitive to anything she took. However, the Vermont winter had been particularly cold and damp, and there was a lot of tumult at her company, Archer Industries, which created more than the usual amount of stress. Dr. Craig prescribed cyclobenzaprine (Flexeril), but after taking a half tablet two hours before bedtime, Sarah felt like a zombie for part of the next day. Dr. Craig changed to nortriptyline (Pamelor), which made her mouth so dry that she had to get up several times during the night to drink water. Next, trazodone (Desyrel) therapy was given, which helped Sarah sleep but did not relieve her painful spasms. Finally, Dr. Craig recommended using liquid doxepin (Sinequan) drops, which made Sarah sleep and relieved her muscle pain and spasms.

Numerous TCA preparations are available to treat fibromyalgia, but as in Sarah's case, it often takes several attempts before the right dose and preparation are found for that individual. *Amitriptyline (Elavil)* can decrease pain, promote restful sleep, and relax muscles in doses of 10–80 mg taken at night. It is the best studied of all the TCAs. A 2008 review of 13 randomized controlled trials demonstrated a mean reduction of pain by 26% and improvement of quality of life by 30%. This is very similar to results noted in the three FDA approved preparations. *Cyclobenzaprine (Flexeril)* is a muscle relaxant without psychotropic properties which promotes restful sleep in doses of 5–30 mg at bedtime. *Doxepin (Sinequan)* is similar to amitriptyline in efficacy and dosing but is also available as a liquid suspension or as a 3 or 6 mg pill in drug sensitive patients who prefer less than 10 mg nightly. Doxepin may induce more weight gain in higher doses. *Nortriptyline, desiprimine* and *imipramine* are similar to amitriptyline, but may be less effective analgesics. They are used in doses of 25 mg to 100 mg at bedtime for analgesics. All of these drugs are better tolerated if they are given several hours before bedtime, and if they are begun at a low dose and escalated very slowly. *Trazodone (Desyrel)* is a heterocyclic compound closely related to TCAs, with fewer side effects and is primarily used as a hypnotic. This can be given in doses of 50–200 mg before retiring. TCAs should be used very carefully, if at all, in young children (under the age of 12), in patients who are pregnant or breast-feeding, and in elderly people who might become confused in the middle of the night. For instance, when older patients are dizzy, sleepy, and have poor balance, they could fall and fracture an osteoporotic hip when they get up to go to the bathroom. Sometimes, the effects of TCAs wear off with time. "Drug holidays," or weeks without using them, or temporarily switching to a different TCA, can restore their effectiveness.

How Much Medication Should a Patient Take and for How Long?

As we've noted, fibromyalgia patients generally don't like to take medicine, and few doctors will prescribe TCAs if patients think they must be taken forever. In fact, this need not be. We usually reevaluate our patients one month after starting a TCA. If their responses are favorable, the TCA is continued in a full dose for three–six months. At that point, we usually taper the drug to every other night and ultimately advise the patient to use it as needed. In other words, when a good night's sleep is critical, when it's been a particularly stressful time, when premenstrual symptoms are present, or if the weather has changed, a few nights on a TCA can be helpful. We have found that several months on a TCA tends to reset one's "pain thermostat," or threshold, and long-term use of the drug is frequently not needed. A summary of several published studies suggests that TCAs alone lead to a significant improvement in one-third of fibromyalgia patients after three months and some improvement in another third after six months of treatment.

Table 22.2. *Medication Families Used for Managing Aspects of Fibromyalgia*

Tricyclic and closely related antidepressant preparations (TCAs)
Amitriptyline hydrochloride (Elavil, Endep)
Imipramine hydrochloride (Janimine, Tofranil)
Doxepin hydrochloride (Adapin, Sinequan)
Nortriptyline hydrochloride (Aventyl, Pamelor)
Desipramine hydrochloride (Norpramin, Petrofane)
Trazodone hydrochloride (Desyrel)
Cyclobenzaprine hydrochloride (Flexeril)

Specific serotonin reuptake inhibitors (SSRIs)
Fluoxetine hydrochloride (Prozac)
Sertraline hydrochloride (Zoloft)
Paroxetine hydrochloride (Paxil)
Citalopram (Celexa)

Combination TCA-SSRI preparations (SNRIs)
Venlafaxine hydrochloride (Effexor)
Nafazodone (Serzone)
Milnacipran (Savella)
Duloxetine (Cymbalta)
Mirtazapine (Remeron)

Dopaminergic agents
L-Dopa (Sinemet)
Ropinerole (Requip)
Pramipexole (Mirapex)

OPIOID receptor antagonist
Naltrexone

Muscle relaxants
Tizanidine (Zanaflex)
Carisoprodol (Soma)
Methocarbamol (Robaxin)
Metaxalone (Skelaxin)

Benzodiazepines and closely related drugs
Clonazepam (Klonopin)
Lorazepam (Ativan)
Diazepam (Valium)
Chlordiazepoxide (Librium)
Alprazolam (Xanax)
Zolpidem (Ambien)
Temazepam (Restoril)
Sodium oxybate (Xyrem)

Anticonvulsants
Lamotrigine (Lamictal)
Topiramate (Topomax)
Carbamazepine (Tegretol),
Levetiracetam (Keppra)
Mexilitine (Mexetil)

Table 22.2. *(Continued)*

Nonsteroidal anti-inflammatory drugs
Salicylates
Aspirin
Sodium salicylates (Trilisate, Disalcid)
Diflusinal (Dolobid)
Magnesium salicylate (Magan, Doan's)

Propionic acid derivatives
Oxaprozin (Daypro)
Naproxen (Naprosyn, Anaprox, Aleve)
Flurbiprofen (Ansaid)
Ibuprofen (Motrin, Advil, Mediprin, Nuprin)
Ketoprofen (Orudis KT, Orudis, Oruvail)
Fenoprofen (Nalfon)
Acetic acid derivatives
Sulindac (Clinoril)
Diclofenac (Voltaren, Cataflam, Arthrotec, Flector)
Tolmetin (Tolectin)
Indomethacin (Indocin)

Selective Cox-2 blockers
Celecoxib (Celebrex)

Others
Meloxicam (Mobic)
Etodolac (Lodine)
Ketrolac (Toradol)
Piroxicam (Feldene)
Nabumetone (Relafen)
Meclofenamate (Meclomen, Ponstel)

Pain Killers
Mild to moderate pain
Acetaminophen (Tylenol)
Tramadol (Ultram, Ultracet)

Moderate to severe pain
Codeine
Oxycodone (Percocet, Percodan), oxycontin, oxymorphone
Hydrocodone (Vicodin, Norco)
Morphine derivatives (numerous)
Dilaudid
Fentanyl
Methadone

Stimulants
Bupropion (Wellbutrin)
Amphetamine salts
Modafinil derivatives (Provigil, Nuvigil)
Cough medicines
Dextromethorphan
Guaifenesin

Atypical antipsychotics
Quetiapine (Seroquel)

Hormones
Growth hormone/pyridostigmine
Melatonin (Ramelton/Rozeram)
Dehydroepiandrosterone (DHEA)

Serotonin Boosters

Selective serotonin reuptake inhibitors (SSRIs) primarily increase levels of serotonin. They include agents such as *fluoxetine (Prozac), paroxetine (Paxil), sertraline (Zoloft)* and the closely related *citalopram* and *escitalopram (Celexa, Lexapro).* None of these agents have analgesic or sleep promoting properties and all clinical studies in FM have had negative results. Since SSRIs may help depression and anxiety, many FM patients are also taking these drugs. The major caveat is that none should be suddenly discontinued because of the possibility of a potentially life-threatening acute "serotonin withdrawal syndrome."

On the other hand, some serotonin containing preparations also have norepinephrine and are useful in fibromyalgia. These include duloxetine and milnacipran, which are approved for use in FM and are discussed above. Patients are cautioned to taper these agents if their use is no longer necessary. *Venlafaxine (Effexor)* and *nafazodone (Serzone)* are ineffective in FM. On the other hand, *mirtazapine (Remeron)* is helpful for sleep issues in patients with significant anxiety.

Dopaminergic Agents

Brain imaging studies have suggested that gray matter regions of the brain have decreased dopamine metabolism. Indeed, agents such as *pramipexole (Mirapex)*, and *ropinirole (Requip)* are D3 receptor agonists approved for use in periodic limb movement syndrome, or restless legs syndrome, which is seen with FM (as well as for Parkinson's syndrome in much higher doses). Several controlled trials have suggested improved scores on assessments of pain, fatigue, function, and global status, especially in narcotic dependent or disabled patients in FM. Anxiety, compulsive or manic behavior, and weight loss may occur.

Naltrexone

Naltrexone is an inexpensive opiate receptor antagonist used in the management of alcohol, opiate, and tobacco dependence and withdrawal. Evidence that it decreases glial cell hyperexcitability led to several FM trials using low doses (4.5 mg daily) suggesting it decreased pain levels by about 30%.

Muscle Relaxants

Tizanidine (Zanaflex) activates alpha-2 adrenergic receptors that control sympathetic nervous system discharges, and some studies have suggested mild efficacy in FM, although there are better data that it has muscle relaxant effects. The usual dose is 4–8 mg at bedtime. *Carisoprodol (Soma), orphenadrine (Norgesic)* and *metaxalone (Skelaxin)* have been prescribed for over 30 years as non-drowsy inducing muscle relaxants (which is untrue) with subjective benefits but they have never had had any positive trial in FM. Significant muscle and nerve spasticity may respond to *dantrolene* or *baclofen*. Some tricyclics (e.g., cyclobenzaprine) and benzodiazepines (e.g., diazepam) are muscle relaxants discussed elsewhere.

Benzodiazepines

Benzodiazepines diminish the alpha-delta wave sleep abnormality, improve sleep myoclonus (restless legs), are FDA approved for anxiety, and inhibit the transmission of excitatory nerve impulses by increasing levels of gamma aminobutyric acid, or GABA, thus acting as muscle relaxants. The National Fibromyalgia Association published an Internet survey in 2007 of 2,596 patients who were asked to list the most perceived effective preparations for the syndrome. Of the top six, three were benzodiazepines (alprazolam, zolpidem, and clonazepam). Despite this, no randomized controlled trial of any benzodiazepine has shown any efficacy. The probable reason is that most of these agents lost their patent protection by the time they were studied, poor trial design, and the fact that sponsors were not interested in funding expensive, well-designed studies for generic preparations. Nevertheless, many practitioners use alprazolam (Xanax) to manage daytime anxiety, lorazepam (Ativan) to treat nighttime anxiety-related insomnia, clonazepam (Klonopin) to promote sleep and muscle relaxation as well as treating restless legs syndrome, diazepam (Valium) for muscle spasm and anxiety, and zolpidem (Ambien) or temazepam (Restoril) to improve sleep. Many are used in combination with other FM agents. All of these preparations are tolerizing (less effective with daily, continuous use) and associated with a withdrawal syndrome when suddenly discontinued. We conclude that benzodiazepines can be prescribed in FM patients when carefully monitored by a knowledgeable primary care physician, rheumatologist, or mental health professional.

Sodium Oxybate (Xyrem)

Sodium oxybate (Xyrem) is a salt of gamma hydroxybutyrate (GHB), a metabolite of gamma alpha butyric acid (GABA). A benzodiazepine-related compound, it is approved for narcolepsy in the United States, Canada, and Europe via a highly restricted supply mechanism. Several large studies have shown that it improves pain and sleep quality in FM patients. Although generally well tolerated, the agent is a liquid that requires the patient being awakened after four hours to take a second dose. It is also closely related to the GHB containing "date rape" drug, rophynol. As a result of these concerns, in 2010 an FDA Advisory Board voted 20–2 not to recommend this drug for FM.

Anticonvulsants

Lamotrigine (Lamictal), topiramate (Topomax), carbamazepine (Tegretol), leve-tiracetam (Keppra) and *mexilitine (Mexetil)* can improve numbness, burning, tingling, depression, anxiety, and headaches associated with FM via sodium or calcium channel blockade and increasing GABA levels. There are no evidence-based studies supporting their use for FM, but many of our patients are prescribed these agents as adjunctive therapies. On the other hand, *gabapentin (Neurontin)* is very similar to pregabalin (see above), and in a single controlled trial results similar to that agent were found. We usually prescribe 100-300 mg at bedtime.

Are NSAIDS (Nonsteroidal Antiinflammatory Drugs), Aspirin or Acetaminophen beneficial?

NSAIDs and aspirin block the actions of a chemical known as *prostaglandin,* which is responsible for some of the pain and inflammation of arthritis. Most fibromyalgia patients are familiar with these preparations, which are listed in Table 22.2. Preparations such as Advil and Aleve are available without a prescription. Most FM patients take NSAIDs on a regular basis for "peripheral" co-occurring sources of musculoskeletal pain such as osteoarthritis or rheumatoid arthritis.

Although these drugs are not dramatically effective in managing fibromyalgia, placebo-controlled double-blinded trials have shown that ibuprofen (the active ingredient of Advil and Motrin) and naproxen (Naprosyn, Aleve, Naprelan) in combination with other fibromyalgia remedies decrease pain in patients with the syndrome. They also alleviate premenstrual syndrome complaints, joint aches, and headaches. Doctors managing fibromyalgia patients recommend that these agents be used in any of several ways. First, they may be used on an occasional as-needed basis for pain breakthroughs. In this instance, blood counts need to be checked once or twice a year. Second, an NSAID may be prescribed on an ongoing, regular basis. In this case, patients should visit their doctor every three to four months and have laboratory testing, including a blood count, and liver and kidney function screening. Third, NSAIDs and salicylates are available topically that can be applied to painful areas (e.g., Voltaren Gel, Flector Patch, Aspercreme, Ben-Gay).

NSAIDs and aspirin are not without side effects. Patients who take these agents on a regular basis may experience fluid retention, bloating, rise in blood pressure, liver or kidney dysfunction, upset stomach, diarrhea, or constipation. Ongoing administration requires checking patients for gastrointestinal ulcers, liver and kidney function, and rashes. In one large survey, in the United States, 10% of regular NSAID users annually had gastric ulcers, or perforations or bleeds, necessitating hospitalization in 3% of regular users. This can be decreased by the use of proton pump inhibitors (e.g., omeprazole [Prilosec]) or intermittent use of these agents.

Pain Killers: From Tylenol to Opiates

Pain killers are analgesics that temporarily deaden the discomfort of fibromyalgia without addressing the reason why patients are in pain, are tired, have difficulty sleeping or are experiencing psychosocial distress. *These agents have little to no use for FM but are widely prescribed, and can be extremely dangerous.* Since higher and higher doses are needed after a while to maintain the same level of effectiveness, many painkillers are addicting. Narcotic preparations tend to be constipating, produce nausea, and reduce mental acuity.

Drugs Marketed for Mild to Moderate Pain

The safest but least effective analgesic is *acetaminophen* (Tylenol). To protect the liver and kidney, patients should never take more than six tablets a day. No study has suggested that acetaminophen (Tylenol, paracetamol) has any effect upon fibromyalgia discomfort.

Tramadol (Ultram) is a novel analgesic with weak agonist activity via the mu opioid receptor and dual serotonin and norepinephrine reuptake inhibition. It has been shown in two randomized controlled trials to be somewhat effective in FM, both alone and in combination with acetaminophen (*Ultracet*). Tramadol is addicting and associated with lowering seizure thresholds.

Drugs Marketed for Moderate to Severe Pain

Allan herniated disks in his neck and low back after a skydiving accident. Although surgery was successful in aligning the spine, he experienced excruciating pain in his neck, low back, and adjacent muscles. Allan consulted neurologists, neurosurgeons, orthopedists, and rheumatologists (two of each). He underwent three MRI scans, two CT scans, an EMG with nerve conduction study, numerous X-rays of his cervical and lumbar spine, and blood tests. Dr. Sand ultimately diagnosed him as having a postsurgical pain amplification syndrome with post-traumatic fibromyalgia. Although Allan looked healthy, without oxycodone (Percodan) and carisoprodol (Soma) he was barely able to move without screaming. Over several months, the amount of Percodan needed to make his life tolerable increased from four to eight pills a day. Dr. Sand referred Allan to a comprehensive pain management center. They admitted him to the hospital and gave him a 72-hour timed release narcotic patch to avoid the problems of withdrawal or craving. He was seen by a physical therapist and an occupational therapist. An anesthesiologist provided local nerve blocks and trigger point injections; a psychologist initiated biofeedback and other relaxation techniques; and a psychiatrist prescribed high doses of a TCA to make him less aware of the pain along with gabapentin (Neurontin). The doctors met for an hour once a week and coordinated Allan's care. After three weeks, he was discharged on tapering doses of medicines and felt better than he had in a long time.

We occasionally prescribe narcotic analgesics for post-surgical pain or short-term use (less than one week for acute flares) or for breakthrough pain (a few tablets a month). *Codeine* is available alone or in combination with either aspirin or acetaminophen but frequently causes nausea. *Hydrocodone* (Vicodin or Norco, with acetaminophen; or vicoprofen, with ibuprofen, Lortab) and *oxycodone* (Percodan, with aspirin; or Percocet, with acetaminophen) are very potent, highly addictive, toxic to the liver and kidney, induce drowsiness, and become less effective with time. Doctors should be on their guard if a patient requests Vicodin with Soma since this combination can produce a dangerous, addictive high and is sold as a street drug.

An increasing problem in clinical practice is that FM patients are placed on opioids, and stay on them for long periods of time despite a lack of documentation of improvement in pain or function. Studies have shown that 15–32% of FM patients in tertiary centers are using these agents. Most of those prescribing these drugs fall into two categories: desperate primary care physicians who are unfamiliar with the intricate aspects of managing FM, and pain centers which address localized pain (e.g., disc disease) with narcotics and nerve blocks without realizing that the patient's pain is chronic and widespread. ***No single controlled study with a high evidence level has shown any efficacy for any opiate in FM.*** Although it can often be very difficult to get these patients off opiates, one approach that can be helpful is to ask the patients if they really feel these drugs are improving their pain, and when they respond negatively as they typically do, then suggest that these drugs be slowly tapered as they are replaced with more efficacious classes of drugs. Basic science work has demonstrated that *opiates promotes glial cell hyperexcitability which leads to the production of cytokines that actually result in increased pain.*

Stronger narcotics are available as a triplicate or "controlled" prescription, whereby copies are sent to state or federal agencies for closer monitoring. Any physician who uses triplicate preparations should have some training in pain management techniques. Many states now require those who prescribe these agents take extra courses in pain management and that chronic narcotic users sign a pain contract. Only a small minority of fibromyalgia patients ever require *morphine, hydromorphine* (Dilaudid), *levorphanol* (Levo-Dromoran), *oxycodone (Percocet, Percodan), fentanyl patches,* or much more expensive brand name preparations (e.g., *Avinza, Kadian, Oromorph*). Another opioid, *methadone,* may additionally block NMDA receptors. In pain management centers, these agents are also available as timed-release patches or in pumps for severe cases. In our experience, some fibromyalgia patients who progress this far also have severe psychiatric disorders or reflex sympathetic dystrophy (see Chapter 13). Opioid receptors become less responsive to actions of the NMDA pathway with time. Fibromyalgia patients with serious pain have the best outcome when they are managed as Allan was at a multidisciplinary pain center employing the coordinated use of pain medications, nerve blocks, counseling, and physical rehabilitation techniques.

Stimulants

There are few agents that have been shown to specifically help improve fatigue in FM. As noted above, the dual reuptake inhibitors such as milnacipran and duloxetine may be helpful in treating this symptom. Weak stimulants such as modafinl (Provigil, Nuvigil) or buproprion (Wellbutrin) may also be useful, although there is little good data supporting this. In our anecdotal experience, the use of more powerful stimulants such as amphetamines and related drugs (e.g., Ritalin, Dexedrine, Addreall) don't have any impact upon pain but can be used as an adjunct in selected patients with specific behaviors where a psychiatrist or mental health professional believes that their use may be appropriate. Older remedies such as vitamin B12 injections, thyroid, and phentermine containing diet pills have no real effect. The latter two can raise heart rates and increase anxiety. One of the best ways to improve fatigue is to promote restful sleep at night and avoid daytime naps.

Expectorants, Antitussives and NMDA Antagonists

Dextromethorphan and *guaifenesin* are components of cough medicines (e.g., Mucinex, Robitussin) that may have mild NMDA antagonist actions. Widely promoted by a single private practice as a fibromyalgia agent, the only controlled trial of guaifenesin outside of the private practice center produced negative results. In view of their widespread use, the study of these agents in an independent setting would be desirable. The NMDA antagonist *ketamine* is too toxic for routine use in FM. In general, the use of NMDA antagonists has been disappointing in pain patients because it appears as though adequately blocking the actions of this receptor leads to too many untoward side effects. Many drugs are in development, however, that act similarly by blocking the activity of glutamate in the CNS.

Cannabinoids (Medical Marijuana)

Medical marijuana has been used by cancer patients to treat nausea and pain. A small single double-blind, placebo-controlled study with nabilone, a drug FDA approved cannabinoid for nausea in cancer, demonstrated significant improvements in the FIQ and pain inventories.

Atypical Antipsychotics

A family of medications known as atypical antipsychotics is widely used for bipolar illness, schizophrenia, anxiety and depression. One of these agents, *quetiapine (Seroquel),* has been evaluated in two controlled studies that showed decreases in the FIQ score and improvement in sleep quality. Since weight gain is common in higher doses, our group prescribes 25–100 mg at bedtime. As noted in Chapter 17, bipolar illness is statistically associated with FM and some of these patients do particularly well with this agent.

Hormonal Approaches

FM patients may have decreased growth hormone levels released during sleep, and approximately one third also have low levels of insulin-like growth factor (IGF-1). There is evidence that GH administration in these FM patients with low IGF-1 led to improvement in a number of symptoms, but this has never been widely used because of the cost and need for intramuscular administration. It is possible that compounds that are being developed that lead to the release of GH and IGF-1 and may be helpful, including older medications such as *pyridostigmine.* Some patients report amelioration of FM symptoms in early menopausal states with hormone replacement therapy. *Melatonin* repairs muscular microtrauma and is available as a supplement and an analog is available as a prescription sleep aid *(Rozeram).* These compounds might have some beneficial effect in FM but have not been extensively studied. *DHEA (dehydroepiandrosterone)* is made by the adrenal gland and is available over the counter and may help fatigue and cognitive dysfunction, but controlled studies in FM were disappointing. Doses of 50–200 mg daily have been used. There have been claims but no evidence that *oxytocin, thymus gland extracts, bromocriptine, calcitonin, colostrum, pregnenolone, thyroid* or *corticosteroids* improve FM.

MISCELLANEOUS AGENTS AND INTERVENTIONS

A potpourri of other interventions has been used in FM and are enumerated below:

- Antibiotics only have potential applications in some FM patients who have gastrointestinal symptoms (see Chapter 13).
- Antiviral medications have been studied in chronic fatigue syndromes without success.
- Antifungal preparations, such as those which treat yeast, are not effective.
- Immunizations are safe in FM but have no influence on the syndrome.
- Allergy shots are safe in FM but have no influence on the syndrome.
- Intravenous immune globulin (IVIG) has slight effects upon fatigue in chronic fatigue syndrome, is prohibitively expensive but has never been studied for FM.

COMPLEMENTARY AND ALTERNATIVE MEDICINE (CAM)

Nearly 30 billion dollars are spent annually in the United States on complementary and alternative medicines, 40% of which represents an out-of-pocket expense. Over 90% of FM patients have used topical agents, massage, chiropractic therapy, homeopathy, acupuncture, or gone on special diets at one time or another, and 40% try at least one approach in any given year. Despite this, very few randomized clinical trials have examined the efficacy of any of these interventions.

CAM treatments and modalities are divided into categories that are enumerated in Table 22.3. Those which work on the mind-body connection, such as meditation, guided imagery, yoga, or other relaxation techniques modulate the autonomic nervous system and tend to be effective in some FM patients. Approaches involving physical efforts (e.g., Pilates, chiropractic) can be useful if proper attention is given to the body mechanics reviewed in Chapter 19. Finally, herbs, vitamins, supplements, and special diets have not been subject to the rigor necessary to demonstrate their usefulness. Sometimes, a sympathetic practitioner who is reassuring can end up helping the patient as much as the supplements as they recommend. Musculoskeletal specialists tend to take a "do no harm" approach when asked about supplements by patients. Since they are not subject to scrutiny by regulatory agencies, these preparations may or may not have the amount of product listed on their label and could have sensitizing preservatives which also interfere with absorption.

TREATING THE MAJOR SYMPTOMS OF FIBROMYALGIA

As can be seen thus far, there are many physical, mental, and pharmacologic approaches that are used for FM. What is the best approach? Which medicines, if any should be prescribed? What symptoms or physical findings warrant what kind of intervention? Table 22.4 summarizes the general thought process that most practitioners who care for FM patients utilize. It involves confirming the diagnosis and other co-existing conditions, as well as educating the patient. This includes recommending exercise, improving coping, and instruction in sleep hygiene. If a specific region of the body is responsible for a significant amount of overall discomfort (e.g., 30% or more), local approaches such as injections or physical measures may be helpful. Medications are tailored to ameliorate sleep, fatigue, psychologic, muscular and pain issues and are reviewed in the next paragraph. Finally, patients with other central sensitization syndromes or autonomic dysfunction may benefit from specific additional interventions. A minority of FM patients report complicated histories that may warrant referral to a pain management center, psychiatrist, or multidisciplinary treatment facility.

Table 22.3. *Examples of Complementary and Alternative Medicine Used for FM That Have Been Critically Evaluated in Peer Review Literature*

Manipulative, physical and manual modalities
Acupuncture *
Alexander technique
Chiropractic
Feldenkrais therapy *
Massage *
Osteopathy
Reflexology
Tai chi*
Yoga
Aerobic training *
Detoxification regimens
Chelation therapy
Colonic irrigation
Magnet therapy

Mental modalities
Aromatherapy
Autogenic training *
Biofeedback *
Cognitive behavioral therapy *
Guided imagery *
Hypnotherapy *
Meditation
Prayer
Spiritual healing

Herbal, dietary and nutriceutical approaches
Magnesium supplements at 500–1000 mg per day
Folk remedies
Naturopathy
Ascorbigen
Co-enzyme Q10
Gingko biloba
Chlorella pyrenoidosa
S-adenosyl methionine *
Vitamins B6, B12, C, D
Echinacea
Evening primrose
L-tryptophan
Peppermint
St John's wort *
Valerian root
Melatonin *

* Controlled studies suggest some benefit.

What Are the Best Medications Used to Manage Poor Sleep?

Sleep is best managing by evaluating the reason for disrupted sleep patterns. The patient should be screened for a history of periodic limb movement syndrome, sleep apnea, use of alcohol or drugs that influence sleep, psychosocial stressors

Table 22.4. *Treatment Approach for Fibromyalgia*

1. Does the patient fulfill criteria for FM?If yes, then:
   a. Consider whether label may be harmful (e.g. in adolescents or in patients with high levels of anxiety about the diagnosis)
   b. Educate the patient about the syndrome
   c. Establish the presence of and address any medical or psychiatric co-morbidities
2. Review non medication treatment modalities such as:
   a. sleep hygiene instruction
   b. principles of exercise
   c. cognitive behavioral therapies such as pacing, relaxation, pleasant activity scheduling, etc.
3. Is the syndrome prominent in a single region of the body?
   a. Assess the usefulness of more local therapies such as injection, topical applications, physical or occupational therapy
4. Is FM affecting the patient's quality of life to the point that medication is indicated? If so, consider the following therapies:
   a. TCAs at bedtime
   b. Pregabalin alone (perhaps for patients with prominent sleep disturbances)
   c. SNRI alone (duloxetine, milnacipran) for patients with co-morbid depression or prominent fatigue
   d. Any of these classes of drugs in a, b, c can be used in combination
   e. Consider using other classes of drugs noted above with less well documented efficacy
5. Address and treat associated central sensitivity syndromes such as tension headache, functional bowel syndrome, chronic pelvic region pain
6. Address and treat autonomic symptoms
7. Consider consultation with a musculoskeletal or pain specialist versed in managing FM, and/or referral to psychiatrist or psychologist to manage co-morbid psychiatric conditions

leading to stress and anxiety, and be instructed in the rules of sleep hygiene reviewed. From a medication standpoint, the following families of drugs tend to be the most effective: tricyclics (especially trazodone, amitriptyline, cyclobenzaprine); SNRIs (especially mirtazapine); benzodiazepines (especially clonazepam, lorazepam, zolpidem); anticonvulsants (especially pregabalin or gabapentin); and melatonin. Many patients use diphenhydramine (Benadryl) because it is available over the counter, but this agent has no real influence upon FM. Restless legs syndrome (15% of all patients) respond to dopaminergic drugs, such as pramipexole as well as iron and clonazepam.

What Are the Best Medications Used to Manage Fatigue?

Once non-FM related sources of fatigue such as infection, anemia, inflammation, hormonal imbalance, depression, malnutrition, malignancy, or pregnancy are ruled out, sleep hygiene should be addressed to ensure that patients sleep well at night and stay up during daytimes. Patients best pace themselves with periods of activity alternating with periods of rest, and implement anxiety reduction and mind-body measures. Medications widely used in FM patients such as milnacipran, fluoxetine, serotonin boosters, and bupropion diminish fatigue. If necessary (or in less than 5% of cases), amphetamine salts (e.g. Ritalin, Dexedrine,

Adderall) can be given short term as they tend to wear off with time. Modafinil and its derivates (Provigil, Nuvigil) are also useful.

What Are the Best Medications Used to Treat FM-Associated Depression and Anxiety?

Counseling should always be the first treatment modality used for FM-associated depression and anxiety. Appropriate practitioners who could be part of the health care team include psychiatrists, psychologists, counselors (e.g., degrees in nursing, social work), clergy, and even mentors or peers in the community. Should medication be desired, TCAs (to promote sleep and diminish depression and anxiety); SNRIs (effective for depression, pain and anxiety); benzodiazepines (for anxiety, sleep, and muscle tightness); SSRIs (for anxiety and depression); anticonvulsants (for anxiety, sleep and pain) alone or in combination with other agents may be useful. If the primary care physician is the prescribing practitioner, periodic consultation with a mental health professional (especially a psychopharmacologist) may additionally be beneficial.

What Is the Optimal Medication Management for Muscle Aches, Spasm, and Stiffness?

Many FM patients have concurrent osteoarthritis or other arthridites and take acetaminophen or nonsteroidal anti-inflammatory agents. Focalized painful tender points or regions of muscle tightness can be approached locally with physical measures, relaxation techniques, topical agents, injections, and exercise. Generalized non-inflammatory systemic aching and spasm responds to agents that promote restful sleep as well as TCAs (particularly cyclobenzaprine), tramadol, and tizanidine. Muscle relaxants (e.g., methocarbamol) are minimally helpful and sedating.

And Finally: What Is the Best Medication Approach for FM Pain?

Patients with FM and pain should undergo a thorough physical examination to ascertain its source. Areas of inflammation, osteoarthritis, mechanical injuries, diabetic nerve or muscle damage or deformities need to be considered separately. It the discomfort is in a classic FM distribution, all the measures listed in the four above paragraphs should be considered. Specifically, FM pain can be ameliorated by anticonsulsants (e.g. pregabalin, gabapentin), acetaminophen with tramadol (e.g., Ultracet), milnacipran, duloxetine, and nonsteroidal anti-inflammatory agents. As mentioned earlier, narcotic analgesics should be avoided if at all possible. Referral to a multidisciplinary pain management program may be appropriate.

Table 22.5. *Remedies Prescribed for Syndromes Associated with FM*

1. Tension headache
   a. Ergot alkaloids
   b. Triptans
   c. Analgesic/caffeine/butalbital combinations (e.g., Fioricet)
   d. Preventive measures with tricyclics, anticonvulsants, beta blockers, SSRIs, calcium channel blockers
2. Irritable bowel and nonulcer dyspepsia
   a. H2 blockers
   b. Proton pump inhibitors
   c. Prokinetic drugs (e.g. metoclopramide)
   d. Antispasmodics (e.g., hyoscamine)
   e. Probiotics
   f. Tricyclics
3. Dysautonomia
   a. Low doses of beta blockers
   b. Clonidine
   c. Fludrocortisone, midrodine for neurally mediated hypotension
4. Dysmenorrhea
   a. NSAIDs
   b. Diuretics
   c. Analgesics
5. Irritable bladder/interstitial cystitis
   a. TCAs
   b. Benzodiazepines
   c. Dimethylsulfoxide
   d. Elmiron

MANAGING ASSOCIATED CENTRAL SENSITIZATION SYNDROMES

I'm very brave generally… only to-day I happen to have a headache.

Lewis Carroll (1832–1898),
Through the Looking Glass 1871

Most FM patients have at least one other central sensitivity syndrome, such as IBS, tension headache, interstitital cystitis, and a number of other conditions. Remedies for specific complaints related to these associated syndromes are frequently used concomitantly with FM medications. A partial listing is summarized in Table 22.5.

FOR FURTHER READING

Arnold LM. Systemic therapies for chronic pain. In: Wallace DJ and Clauw DJ. eds. Fibromyalgia and other central pain syndromes. Philadelphia: Lippincott Williams & Wilkins, 2005, pp. 365–388.

Arnold LM, Clauw DJ, Dunegan LJ, Turk DC. A framework for fibromyalgia management for primary care providers. *Mayo Clin Proc* 2012; *87*: 488–496.

Arthritis Foundation. *Guide to Alternative Therapies*. J. Horstman (Editor). Atlanta, Georgia: Arthritis Foundation, 1999.

Berman BM, Swyers JP. Complementary medicine treatments for fibromyalgia syndrome. *Ballieres Best Clin Prac Res Clin Rheumatol* 1999; *13*: 487–492.

Bernardy K, Fuber N, Killner, Hause W. Efficacyof cognitive-behavioral therapies in fibromyalgia syndrome—A systemic review and metaanalysis of randomized controlled trials. *J Rheumatol* 2010; *37*: 1991–2005.

Boomershine CS, Crofford LJ. A symptom-based approach to pharmacologic management of fibromyalgia. *Nature Reviews Rheumatology* 2009; *5*: 191–199.

Busch AJ, Schacter CL, Overend TJ. *et al*. Exercise for fibromyalgia: A systemic review, *J Rheumatol* 2008; *35*: 1130–1144.

Choy E, Marshall D, Gabriel ZI, *et al*. A systemic review and mixed treatment comparison of the efficacy of pharmacological treatments for fibromyalgia. *Semin Arthritis Rheum* 2011; *41*: 335–345.

Crofford LJ, Rowbotham MC, Mease PJ, Russell IJ, Dworkin RH, Corbin AE, Young JP Jr, LaMoreaux LK, Martin SA, Sharma U. Pregabalin 1008-105 Study Group, Pregabalin for the treatment of fibromyalgia syndrome: Results of a randomized, double-blind, placebo-controlled trial. *Arthritis Rheum.* 2005; *52*: 1264–1273.

Hauser W, Bartram-Wunn E, Bartram C. *et al*. Placebo responders in randomized controlled drug trials of fibromyalgia: Systemic review and meta-analysis. *Der Schmerz* 2011; *25*: 619–631.

Holman AJ. Treatment of fibromyalgia: A changing of the guard. *Women's Health* 2005; *1*: 409–420.

Meyer HP. Myofascial pain syndrome and its suggested role in the pathogenesis and treatment of fibromyalgia syndrome. *Curr Pain Headache Rep.* 2002, *6*: 274–283.

Wang C, Schmid CH, Rones R, *et al*. A randomized trial of Tai Chi for fibromyalgia, *N Engl J Med* 2010; *363*: 743–754.

23

The Economic Burden of Fibromyalgia: Work and Disability

Fibromyalgia patients are not disabled; they are differently abled.
Adapted from
James McGuire, M.D. (1949–1997),
rheumatologist

While many initiatives have scrutinized the financial impact of chronic pain, other than back pain, few studies have addressed the economic burden of musculoskeletal pain, or FM per se on society. Most of the published surveys in this area concern themselves with disability.

THE ECONOMIC BURDEN OF FIBROMYALGIA

Chronic pain costs $600 billion a year in the United States, half of which represents musculoskeletal pain. In the mid-1990s, a congressional committee estimated the direct and indirect costs of FM in the United States was somewhere between $12 and $14 billion (which would now be about $20 billion) a year. This includes approximately 10 million office visits in the United States to physicians for pain. The cost of diagnosing fibromyalgia is approximately $6,555, which is largely accounted for by failure of a primary care physician to make the correct diagnosis, excess numbers of office visits, diagnostic testing, and unsuccessful treatment interventions. Canadian data suggested that the annual health insurance costs for FM patients were double those in non-FM beneficiaries. A 2007 United States survey reported that healthcare costs were triple that of non-FM beneficiaries, largely due to high levels of comorbidities and health care utilization. Surprisingly, the annual cost of treating an FM patient in the United States is the same as treating one with rheumatoid arthritis.

THE ECONOMIC IMPACT OF FIBROMYALGIA UPON PRODUCTIVITY AND DISABILITY

It is believed that our nation's productivity is 1–2% less due to FM. Half of all lost work productivity time in the United States is due to depression. In a sampling of 28,902 workers over a two-week period, 13% lost productive work due to pain. Fibromyalgia complaints accounted for one-sixth of this (the most common cause was headache). In Finland, an employed FM patient has a 1.4–1.5 risk for a medically certified absence due to sickness not accounted for by coexisting psychiatric illness, rheumatoid arthritis or psychiatric disorders. Pre-existing psychosocial factors can predict the development of new-onset widespread pain after being hired for a physical job. These include low job satisfaction, low social support, and monotonous work.

DISABILITY

Most of us have to work for a living. There are bills to pay and families to provide for. Since fibromyalgia patients do not usually look ill and on superficial examination appear strong, complaints of difficulty performing the job can be hard to believe. This chapter will review definitions as they apply to disability, impairments reported in fibromyalgia patients, and constructive approaches that allow individuals with the syndrome to work most effectively.

LET'S COME TO TERMS: WHAT IS DISABILITY?

The World Health Organization defines *disability* as a limitation of function that compromises the ability to perform an activity within a range considered normal. Efforts to manage work disabilities considers issues such as age, sex, level of education, psychological profile, past attainments, motivation, retraining prospects, and social support systems. Additionally, work disability issues take into account work-related self-esteem, motivation, stress, fatigue, personal value systems, and availability of financial compensation.

An *impairment* is an anatomic, physiologic, or psychological loss that leads to disability. Impairments include pain from work activities (e.g., heavy lifting), emotional stress (e.g., working in a complaint department), or muscle dysfunction (e.g., cerebral palsy). A *handicap* is a job limitation or something that cannot be done (e.g., deafness).

Patients with a disability can be *permanently, totally disabled* and thus potentially eligible for Social Security Disability and Medicare health benefits. Other classifications include being *permanently, partially disabled,* whereby vocational rehabilitation, occupational therapy, and psychological or ergonomic evaluations can address impairments or handicaps to optimize employment retraining possibilities. *Temporary, partial disability* allows one to work with restrictions (e.g., no lifting more than ten pounds) while treatment is in progress. *Temporary, total disability* involves a leave of absence from employment while undergoing treatment so that one can return to work.

Subjective factors of disability include symptoms such as pain or fatigue, while objective factors of disability are physical signs such as a heart murmur or a swollen joint. One can be disabled from a *work category* and granted disability even if employment is ongoing in a different work category. Work categories are rated as sedentary, light work, light medium work, medium work, heavy work, or very heavy work, each defined by how much exertion is used over a time interval. Additional consideration is given to repetitive motions such as bending, squatting, walking up stairs, and squeezing, as well as environmental temperature or the operating of heavy equipment.

DO MOST FIBROMYALGIA PATIENTS WORK?

In the United States, up to 90% of fibromyalgia patients who wish to work are able to do so. Sixty percent of fibromyalgia patients are working full time. (The other 30% are housewives, househusbands, and retirees.) In a seven-university center study of 1,500 individuals with fibromyalgia, 25% had received disability payments at some time, and 15% received Social Security Disability (and Medicare) benefits. As noted before, studies from university medical centers include patients who have more severe problems and do not reflect the patient population seen in community-based rheumatology practices. Despite this, two-thirds of academic-based study patients related that they were able to work nearly all the time.

However, these statistics are deceiving and do not relate the problems fibromyalgia patients have had with employment. Half report difficulty keeping their job. For example, in another survey, 30% of these patients had to change their jobs due to the disorder, and 30% modified their jobs in some way to accommodate their symptoms. All told, in the United States at any time, 6–15% of employed fibromyalgia patients are on some form of disability costing $10 billion a year in benefits and lost productivity. In nations with more generous disability systems such as Sweden, up to 25% of these patients are considered disabled. FM patients have double the chance of going on disability compared to those without it, and have three times the risk of losing their job.

WHY ARE SOME FIBROMYALGIA PATIENTS DISABLED?

The most common reason fibromyalgia patients say they cannot work is severe pain. This creates many problems because pain is a subjective sensation that is hard for others to understand. After all, employers point out, other employees with pain are able to work. Additional factors that limit employment in fibromyalgia patients include poor cognitive functioning (inability to think clearly), fatigue, stress, and cold, damp work environments. Fibromyalgia patients complain of having decreased stamina or endurance and frequently have poor body mechanics. This limits their ability to undertake repetitive lifting, bending, or squatting, assume unnatural positions, or use excessive force. Using standardized test measurements in a study of light to medium jobs that required repetitive movements, fibromyalgia patients performed only 58.6% of the work done by healthy co-workers. This may be due to a decrease of up to one-third in muscle strength per unit for repetitive activities in patients with the syndrome. Interestingly, there is a discrepancy between perceived work ability and what is viewed on videos of work performance. Most fibromyalgia patients perform better than they think.

Another important factor relates to psychological makeup. Patients unable to deal with pain, low self-esteem, a strong feeling of helplessness, and low educational levels have a worse outlook.

Do fibromyalgia patients malinger, or make up their symptoms for purposes of secondary (such as monetary) gain? Although offers of financial compensation are always attractive, several studies have shown that over 90% of the time, fibromyalgia does not stop after litigation is settled. In Israel, where work disability is not recognized, trauma is associated with the same prevalence of post-injury fibromyalgia as in the United States. On the other hand, an epidemic of fibromyalgia-related "repetitive strain disorder" in the late 1980s in Australia was eliminated by minor changes in regulations.

Who Is Responsible for Disability?

Disability must take into account predisposing factors (e.g., stressful life events, personality, chronic medical illnesses); precipitating factors (e.g., infection, trauma, emotional stress); and perpetuating factors (e.g., not liking work, untreated psychiatric illnesses). Unfortunately, these are rarely the fault of the employer, but in a Worker's Compensation system, all too often the employer is left holding the bag.

WHAT RIGHTS DOES A FIBROMYALGIA PATIENT HAVE?

The Americans with Disabilities Act protects individuals from job discrimination by requiring companies with more than 15 employees to make adjustments ("reasonable accommodations") for people with disabilities and chronic illnesses. These modifications include having an occupational therapist or ergonomic expert evaluate the work site. If fibromyalgia is brought on or aggravated by poor body mechanics or emotional stress caused at work, individuals are eligible for medical treatment, disability, and job retraining through the workers compensation system. Accommodations include part-time or half-day employment or a leave of absence. Most medium-sized and large companies have private disability policies. Although these approaches are all too often abused, their intent is to keep disabled people employed. If the disability is total and permanent, many individuals are eligible for Social Security benefits. Fibromyalgia, however, is not considered a disabling condition by the U.S. government. Therefore, the small number of patients with fibromyalgia who are totally, permanently disabled are usually granted Social Security benefits on the basis of related conditions such as chronic fatigue, pain, arthritis, or depression—all accepted disabilities under government rules.

HOW CAN TOTAL DISABILITY BE PREVENTED?

Vicki was a crack systems analyst whose computer skills got her jobs, but she never seemed able to keep them. Over a five-year period, Vicki had accepted but had been terminated or resigned from five separate positions. She had a long-standing diagnosis of fibromyalgia, which was adequately controlled with a combination of cyclobenzaprine (Flexeril) in the evening and sertraline (Zoloft) in the morning. Vicki encountered numerous problems in trying to hold her jobs: an inability to work overtime when certain projects demanded it, feeling faint when co-workers smoked around her, dealing with terrible chairs and glare at her computer workstations, snickers from co-workers when she took midday breaks, disputes with her boss when she tried to get time off to see her doctor, and being forced to lift 20-pound file boxes. Vicki became defensive, and a bad attitude got her fired from her last job before she completed the probation period. Through her fibromyalgia support group, Vicki was put in contact with an occupational therapist who consulted part-time on workstation ergonomics for a Fortune 500 company. With the help of the occupational therapist and a vocational rehabilitation counselor, Vicki put together a resume showing how productive her work could be and the potential benefits for the company that exploited her creative talents. At her next job interview, Vicki appeared very positive but made it clear that the potential employer would have to recognize her partial disability. By making a few minor modifications to her work schedule, alterations that involved no cost to the company, she could become an outstanding worker. Vicki has now held her job for three years, loves every minute of it, and recently was promoted.

Despite all that has been related in this chapter, almost 90% of fibromyalgia patients in the United States who wish to work can be employed in some capacity. In this section, we'll review strategies that enable patients to minimize pain and function as productively as possible.

Find an Agreeable Environment

Try to find a workplace that is quiet and smoke-free, has clean air or is well ventilated, is adequately lit, heated, and has a comfortable noise level.

Be Up Front and Positive with Your Employer

If fibromyalgia alters work performance or may require workstation or workplace modifications, let the employer know about the syndrome but do it in a positive way. Relate all the things you *can* do and how your productivity can be enhanced with minimal accommodations.

Pace Yourself

Learn to manage time and prioritize job responsibilities and obligations. Make sure that a workday has several rest periods and a reasonable lunch break, which helps minimize fatigue. Focus your energy on what is important. Have a positive attitude and learn to laugh.

Strategize and Use Coping Skills

Co-workers should be made aware of whatever adaptations are necessary for optimal productivity so that they will not view these as perks or become jealous. Learn to cope with the office environment—you cannot fire the boss. Don't get stressed out about what cannot be changed or about policies you do not control.

Examine the Workstation

It is important to limit or avoid excessive lifting, reaching, twisting, standing, bending, overhead use of arms, and squatting. Consider using supportive braces or bands when engaging in these activities. Alternatively, follow employee manuals or physician or allied health professional (e.g., physical or occupational therapist) instructions if these motions are necessary for the job, since it's necessary to minimize harm from work trauma.

Make sure your chair has a firm back and does not compress the circulation. Its height and back should be comfortable and at the right level for your computer keyboard. If the job requires heavy telephone use, consider using a speakerphone or headset to minimize neck and upper back strain. Some individuals perform their work activities better if they wear a back brace, rotate jobs, use rubber mats if prolonged standing is required, and are able to park closer to their office.

Follow the recommendations in the computer manual regarding height, monitor angle, type of chair to be used, and screen glare. Keep arms parallel to hips, the hands above the keyboard and even or below the elbows, wrists straight, and fingers curved; special keyboards or soft pads may be helpful. When typing, arms should hang comfortably from the shoulders. The shoulder should be relaxed and not scrunched. An example is shown in Figure 23.1.

Help Yourself

Maintain correct posture to ease muscle strain, learn to relax, and keep physically conditioned. Take short work breaks to deep-breathe, relax, and stretch. Patients who have difficulty coping or who notice worsening pain shouldn't keep things to themselves. Call a doctor, mental health advisor, or physical therapist.

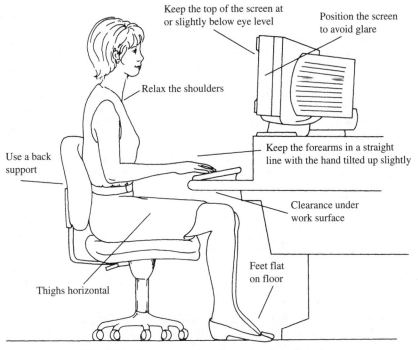

Keep the top of the screen at or slightly below eye level

Position the screen to avoid glare

Relax the shoulders

Use a back support

Keep the forearms in a straight line with the hand tilted up slightly

Clearance under work surface

Feet flat on floor

Thighs horizontal

Fig. 23.1. *An ergonomically correct workstation.*

WHAT'S WRONG WITH OUR CURRENT DISABILITY SYSTEM?

There is no question that our disability system is deeply flawed; nevertheless, we have to operate within it. Why should fibromyalgia patients be excluded from disability eligibility just because of '"bad" systems? In the United States, one's disability is handled through Worker's Compensation, a private disability system, Social Security, or automobile insurance. Since there are no routinely used blood tests for fibromyalgia, a lot of examiners think that some patients "fake" the syndrome. However, fibromyalgia is no different than phantom limb or migraine headaches, which everybody acknowledges are highly subjective, real, and compensable and without specific tests to gauge their severity. The stigmatization of fibromyalgia by caregivers and disability carriers is partly due to the failure to develop adequate tools for assessing fibromyalgia disability; this should not be blamed on the patient. For example, we frequently receive a disability form with queries such as "Can the patient lift ten pounds, always, never, or occasionally?" This may be fine for a stroke patient, but cannot apply to a fibromyalgia patient who at certain days can lift ten pounds, but then for only ten minutes an hour. This is not a problem with the patient. Simply stated, the form was not devised to reflect one's true abilities. Although many of the measurements reviewed to evaluate new drug therapies in Chapter 21 have been tried

Table 23.1. *Disability in FM Summary Points*

1. Fibromyalgia is responsible for a decrease in U.S. productivity by 1–2% and results in direct and indirect expenditures of at least $15 billion a year.
2. 90% of FM patients who wish to are working full time. 10–25% of working FM patients received disability payments at some time, and 40% have changed jobs or job descriptions due to the syndrome.
3. 10% with FM are permanently totally disabled, usually due to inability to deal with severe pain or fatigue or cognitive dysfunction. Most had a history of low self-esteem, anxiety, depression, low educational attainment pre-employment. True work-induced disability is very rare.
4. Methods of work ability ascertainment for FM are lacking, and current metrics are not valid for the syndrome.
5. Patient education, rehabilitation, work station ergonomic assistance can keep most at-risk FM patients in the workforce, and individuals who are given total disability usually deteriorate psychologically and functionally.

to assess disability, they have generally failed. The overwhelming majority of fibromyalgia patients benefit from physical therapy, occupational therapy, vocational rehabilitation, ergonomic workstation assessments, educational sessions, counseling, and medication.

Unfortunately, the current system is insensitive to many of the considerations listed above and leads to more people not working than it should. This does not mean that the system should never compensate for fibromyalgia; it needs improvement. The reason why 10% with fibromyalgia are permanently disabled is rarely the fault of the employer. The system needs to be changed so that these individuals receive treatment, and if necessary, Social Security disability as opposed to work-related disability.

SUMMING UP

The overwhelming majority of patients with fibromyalgia are able to work full time, but up to 40% may have to change jobs or make modifications in order to be productively employed. These individuals may take advantage of existing disability laws, protections, and medical resources to achieve this. The 5–10% of fibromyalgia patients who are totally, permanently disabled usually have severe problems with pain, fatigue, coping skills, or depression.

FOR FURTHER READING

Al-Allaf AW. Work disability and health care utilization in patients with fibromyalgia syndrome. *J Clin Rheumatol* 2007; *13*: 199–201.
Berger A, Dukes E, Martin S, Edelsberg J, Oster G. Characteristics and healthcare costs of patients with fibromyalgia. *International Journal of Clinical Practice*, 2007; *61*: 1498–1508.

Harkness EF, Macfarlane GJ, Nahit E, Silman AJ, Mc Beth J. Mechanical injury and psychosocial factors in the workplace predict the onset of widespread body pain. *Arthritis Rheum* 2005; *50*: 1655–1664.

Hughes G, Martinez C, Myon E, *et al.* The impact of a diagnosis of fibromyalgia on health care resource use by primary care patients in the UK. An observational study based on clinical practice. *Arthritis & Rheumatism* 2006; *54*: 1770–1183.

Silverman S, Dukes EM, Johnston SS, *et al.* The economic burden of fibromyalgia: comparative analysis with rheumatoid arthritis. *Curr Medical Res & Opinion* 2009; *25*: 829–840.

Wallace DJ. *The economic impact of fibromyalgia on society and disability issues, Fibromyalgia and Other Central Pain Syndromes*. In: Wallace DJ and Clauw DJ, eds. Philadelphia: Lippincott Williams & Wilkins, 2005; 395–400.

Wallace DJ, Hallegua DS. Quality-of-life, legal-financial and disability issues in fibromyalgia. *Current Pain Headache Reports* 2001; *5*: 313–319.

White KP, Speechley M, Harth M, Ostbye T. Comparing self-reported function and work disability in 100 community cases of fibromyalgia syndrome versus controls in London, *Ontario, Arthritis Rheum 42*, 1999: 76–83.

White LA, Robinson RL, Yu AP, *et al.* Comparison of health care use and costs in newly diagnosed and established patients with fibromyalgia, *Journal of Pain* 2009; *10*: 976–983.

Part VII
WHERE ARE WE HEADED?

We're the first to agree that the fibromyalgia therapies reviewed in the previous two sections are far from perfect. However, they are a long way from "You'll just have to learn to live with it" advice most doctors offered just a few years ago. The good news is that there are a lot of developments on the horizon. This part discusses the outcomes of fibromyalgia and presents a baseline from which physicians and researchers are working toward improvements. Many new approaches for treating fibromyalgia are the focus of well-designed studies, some of which will make substantial differences in the quality of life for fibromyalgia patients in the near future.

24

What's the Prognosis?

Diseases desperate grown. By desperate appliances are relieved.
Or not at all.

William Shakespeare (1564–1616),
Hamlet, Act 4, Sc. 3, 1. 9

When patients are diagnosed with fibromyalgia, one of their first questions to us relates to its outcome. "Is there hope, doc?" and "Will the pain ever go away?" are two of the more common queries we hear. Unfortunately, few surveys have addressed this issue, and some have arrived at contradictory conclusions. This chapter will try to put these studies in their proper perspective. Yes, there is hope!

WHAT HAPPENS TO MYOFASCIAL PAIN SYNDROME?

When discomfort is limited to a specific region of the body and is not widespread, the outlook for long-term relief of pain is usually quite good. With local physical measures, injections, emotional support, and anti-inflammatory and analgesic medication, as well as instruction in proper body mechanics, over 75% of regional myofascial pain syndrome patients have substantial pain relief within two–three years. Unfortunately, there is little middle ground. For example, in an 18-year analysis of 53 patients with low back pain followed by musculoskeletal specialists, 25% ultimately developed fibromyalgia. Therefore, we believe that myofascial pain should not be shrugged off or given short shrift. A problem that is addressed early and effectively saves patients, health plans, and society money. Also ameliorated are the heartaches of patients and those close to them. Improved productivity promotes a feeling of relief, as well as a better quality of life. When a practitioner prescribes Advil and says that this is all that can be done for TMJ dysfunction syndrome, it is penny wise but pound foolish.

WHAT HAPPENS TO FIBROMYALGIA?

The outcome of fibromyalgia depends on who sees the patient and calls the shots. For example, in one report that tracked family practitioners, internists, or other primary care physicians familiar with fibromyalgia's diagnosis and management, 24% of patients were in remission at two years and 47% no longer met the ACR criteria for the syndrome. This implies that early intervention by a knowledgeable community physician is the first line of therapy. Children with fibromyalgia also have a favorable outcome. In the largest study to date, symptoms resolved in 73% within two years of diagnosis.

The outlook in tertiary care settings is not as rosy. Once the symptoms and signs of the syndrome are serious enough to warrant referral to an academically oriented rheumatologist who is involved in fibromyalgia research, improvement is common but recovery rare. A summary of academic-based studies suggests that at three years, 90% of patients still have symptoms. They were rated as moderate to severe in 60% of the cases, and only 2% were cured. Among these patients, measures of pain, disability, function, fatigue, sleep, and psychological health change disappointingly little over the years. Those who fulfill the criteria for chronic fatigue syndrome tend to get better if they can trace their disease onset to an infection. Among this grouping, two-thirds are improved at two years. In community rheumatology practices, we frequently find that most patients feel better after they are educated about the syndrome and treated. Many generally do well, but if the weather changes, a new emotionally stressful situation occurs, or physical trauma is sustained, relapse may occur. However, since these patients are connected to a rapid-response medical environment, long-term damage or disability can be prevented.

CAN A BAD OUTCOME BE PREDICTED?

Several investigators have tried to find unifying characteristics of patients who failed to respond to treatment. These individuals tended to have severe mood or behavioral disturbances, received less than 12 years of formal education, had poor insight into the sources of psychosocial stressors or were older than 40 when their symptoms began. In our experience, patients who are psychotic (those who carry the diagnosis of schizophrenia, bipolar disease, paranoia, or delusional disorder) or are not successfully treated for substance abuse do not improve. A longitudinal study of 1,555 fibromyalgia patients followed up to 11 years at tertiary centers showed 40% improved over a five-year period. Severity increased in 36% and only 10% had substantial improvement.

WHAT CAN PATIENTS DO TO IMPROVE THEIR OUTLOOK?

In the United States, too many health plans provide too much "tough love." As a result, fibromyalgia patients must be their own advocates. Patients with the syndrome should seek a practitioner who knows what fibromyalgia is, believes that it exists, and wants to help people with the disorder. If a health plan restricts access to this type of physician, patients should reiterate that nearly all health plans are required to provide the best possible care for specific problems. If this care is not available within a certain environment, the insurer must make accommodations to do the best for the subscriber's health and well-being. We're not talking about breaking the bank! A six-center survey of 538 chronic fibromyalgia patients treated in an academic setting (and, by definition, having more severe disease) had an average medical bill of $2,274 a year over a seven-year period. Fibromyalgia patients rarely benefit from surgery or hospitalization for their condition. With the assistance of their fibromyalgia caregiver, patients may need to supply their carrier with evidence supporting the need for physical therapy, occupational therapy, vocational rehabilitation, cognitive therapy, or psychological counseling in order for their symptoms to improve. Patients can help themselves further by joining the Arthritis Foundation, subscribing to fibromyalgia support group newsletters, and keeping abreast of advances in the field. Informed, motivated patients who help themselves ultimately feel better and have an improved quality of life.

THE BOTTOM LINE

If fibromyalgia is identified early and managed appropriately, patients usually improve. Patients who know what fibromyalgia is and are motivated to improve their condition fare better than passive individuals who get lost in the bureaucracy of our medical establishment. In our experience, it's harder for patients to improve (though not impossible) if therapy is delayed for more than five years. Individuals who are psychotic, demonstrate poor insight into their sources of psychosocial distress (if any), or who are addicted to drugs or alcohol, will not improve until their psychiatric and emotional problems are addressed first.

FOR FURTHER READING

Baumgartner E, Finchk A, Cedraschi C, *et al*. A six-year prospective study of a cohort of patients with fibromyalgia. *Ann Rheum Dis* 2002; *61*: 644–645.

Granges G, Zilko P, Littlejohn GO. Fibromyalgia syndrome: Assessment of the severity of the condition two years after diagnosis. *J Rheumatol 21*, 1994: 523–529.

Kennedy M, Felson DT. A prospective long-term study of fibromyalgia syndrome. *Arthritis Rheum 39*, 1996: 682–685

L'apossy E, Maleitzke R, Hycaj P, Mennet P, Muller W. The frequency of transition of chronic low back pain to fibromyalgia. *Scand J Med 24*, 1995: 29–33.

MacFarlane GJ, Thomas E, Papageorgiou AC, Scholum J, Croft PR, Silman AJ. The natural history of chronic pain in the community: A better prognosis than in the clinic? *J Rheumatol 23*, 1996: 1617–1620.

Walitt B, Fitzcharles M-A, Hassett AL, *et al.* A longitudinal outcome of fibromyalgia: A study of 1555 patients. *J RHeumatol* 2011; *38*: 2238–2246.

Wolfe F, Anderson J, Harkness D, Bennett RM, Caro XJ, Goldenberg DL, Russell IJ, Yunus M. B. Health status and disease severity in fibromyalgia: results of a six-center longitudinal study. *Arthritis Rheum 40*, 1997: 1571–1579.

25
The Future Holds a Lot of Hope

The future has waited long enough; If we do not grasp it, other hands, grasping hard and bloody, will.

Adlai Stevenson (1900–1965) to Murray Kempton, 1963

When we became interested in fibromyalgia over 30 years ago, we quickly learned how it felt to be lonely. The Fibrositis Study Club (now the Fibromyalgia Study Club) of the American Rheumatism Association (now the American College of Rheumatology) had an average attendance of ten at its annual meetings. In 2010, more than 1,000 rheumatologists attended the same meeting. During the early 1980s, an average of 14 articles a year appeared in the fibromyalgia medical literature, and less than $100,000 was being spent annually on fibromyalgia research. The recognition of fibromyalgia by organized medicine as a distinct syndrome has had a salutary effect on research. As of this writing, over 1,000 articles are now published yearly and $20 million is spent annually on research. All this attention and interest bodes well for more scientific breakthroughs in the field. What can fibromyalgia patients hope for over the next 20 years?

AN IMPROVED CLASSIFICATION

In all probability, the name *fibromyalgia* will be replaced by a more all-encompassing term, one that includes related syndromes that have similar causes and physiologic processes. A better (and catchier) term that combines symptoms and signs reported in tension headache, pain amplification, irritable bowel syndrome, irritable bladder, and chronic fatigue syndrome, among others, will be devised and agreed on. When organized medicine marshals the resources of experts in gastroenterology, infectious disease, rheumatology, and other subspecialties to work together, our knowledge of pain amplification, neurotransmitter-mediated, behaviorally influenced fatigue syndromes will be increased, and research strategies will be better coordinated and focused. Fibromyalgia advocacy groups will unite to increase funding for research and education that will make a difference.

We predict that 2–5% of the U.S. population has chronic widespread neuro-muscular pain with the systemic overlay mentioned above.

Over the next 20 years, the precise racial and ethnic backgrounds of these individuals will be identified, as well as the genes that influence the process. Additionally, environmental and occupational factors that cause or aggravate chronic neuromuscular pain will be clarified. Through coordinated strategies involving all forms of media, the public will become aware of what fibromy-algia is and what factors are associated with it. Increased awareness through an updated medical education curriculum will allow health care practitioners to intervene earlier to treat patients who develop fibromyalgia symptoms or signs after an injury or infection. This, in turn, will improve the prognosis and out-come. Better support systems will be available for individuals who require all forms of counseling or job retraining through the Arthritis Foundation and fibro-myalgia support organizations.

BASIC RESEARCH ADVANCES

In the next decade, we predict that the body's pain pathways will be better demarcated and understood. Feedback loops and the source of what stimulates or suppresses certain "wires" or nerves will be elucidated. The roles of substance P, serotonin, the ANS, epinephrine, endorphin, dopamine, and other important chemicals that affect mood, pain perception, and transmission of information from one region to another will be better defined. For example, if we can block messages sent by excitatory amino acids (which amplify chronic pain but play no role in acute pain), a new class of drugs that specifically treats fibromyalgia pain can be formulated.

The nervous system does not work in a vacuum but involves interactions with hormones, the immune system, muscles, sleep, and stress factors. The biology of cytokines and other groups of chemicals that interrelate these components will be better understood. Along these lines, investigators will be able to answer several important questions in the next 20 years. Why are some behavior patterns associ-ated with pain amplification but not others? Does muscle spasm result from a local reflex or does it come from signals within the spinal column? What does sleep have to do with growth hormone? Is there anything wrong with the immune sys-tem of fibromyalgia patients? Why do reflexes within the ANS increase numbness, tingling, flushing, headaches, cramping, and burning rather than help people with fibromyalgia? How do viruses or other microbes cause chronic fatigue syndrome? What really goes on inside a local tender point? What do glial cells do in the brain? How does sensory afferent pain processing really work?

PHYSICAL AND PSYCHOLOGICAL INTERVENTIONS

Coordinated efforts will improve physician education and lead to diagnostic testing or imaging that will provide practitioners with readily available tools or "biomarkers" to confirm the diagnosis of fibromyalgia. Skeptical health care professionals will no longer refer to fibromyalgia as a "wastebasket" diagnosis or the "emperor's new clothes" disease. Once a diagnosis is confirmed, our non-medication approaches will be fine-tuned. For example, as more allied health professionals are trained in cognitive therapy, fibromyalgia patients will be able to think better and function with greater mental clarity. Information about physical therapy measures that are harmful in fibromyalgia but useful in other forms of musculoskeletal disease will be better disseminated once more therapists take an Arthritis Foundation certification course detailing specific approaches that do and do not benefit fibromyalgia patients. Exercise and conditioning programs currently being developed will be tested, widely available, and reimbursed by third-party carriers. Ergonomics will play a greater role in the prevention of fibromyalgia as companies find that it is in their interest to have healthy, productive, motivated, pain-free employees working at comfortable workstations. The next editions of the *Diagnosis and Statistical Manual for Mental Disorders (DSM)*, used for psychiatric diagnosis, will confront the chronic neuromuscular pain directly and create a new category for pain amplification. In turn, emphasis will be put on how to diminish psychosocial distress, improve self-esteem, decrease pain perception, and deal with the reactive depression and anxiety related to fibromyalgia. This information will be incorporated into the training of mental health professionals (e.g., psychologists, social workers, counselors, clergy, psychiatrists).

FIBROMYALGIA THERAPIES: THE NEXT GENERATION

Current medications used to manage fibromyalgia will be improved. Newer, less toxic NSAIDs will be on the market in the next few years. Safer and more specific TCAs (e.g., Elavil-like) and SSRI (e.g., Prozac-like) agents are on the horizon. Benzodiazepines (e.g., Klonopin-like) with less potential for inducing depression or addiction will be introduced. Vaccines against fibromyalgia-inducing infections may become available.

New classes of medicines will block substance P (e.g., Pregabalin, nerve growth factor); increase serotonin or adenosine A; release more endorphins; modulate calcium-magnesium in muscle channels or sodium channel blockers in cells; and block excitatory amino acids, nerve growth factor, and dynorphins. Agents that stabilize the ANS will be developed as our knowledge of cell signaling and cell surface receptors evolves. Biochemistry and neurochemistry advances will allow for the development and introduction of medications that act as kinin receptor antagonists, nitric oxide synthetase receptor antagonists, and tachykinin receptor antagonists and analogues of capsaicin. We may wish to augment or block certain cytokines. Thus, any drug that acts as an agonist or antagonist of neurotransmitters might be effective in treating at least a subset of FM patients who develop heightened pain sensitivity in part because of this

Table 25.1. *Template, or Categories for New Drug Development in Fibromyalgia*

1. Chemicals in the *ascending* pain tracts which could influence fibromyalgia
   NMDA blockers
   Nerve growth factor blockers
   Substance P blockers
   Ion channel modulator of sodium, calcium, and magnesium
   Dynorphin blockers
   Serotonin
   Neurotensin
   Cystokinase
2. Chemicals in the *descending* pain tracts which could influence fibromyalgia
   Opiates
   Serotonin
   Dopamine
   Norepinephrine
   GABA
   Adenosine
   Anti-nicoceptive pathways
3. Chemicals that influence cerebral function subject to modification
   Cytokines
   Autonomic nervous system components
   Limbic kindling blockers
   Hormones
4. Anti-inflammatory approaches
5. Topical or local regimens which block limited or regional pain
6. Agents which modulate muscle metabolism
   Hormones
   Muscle relaxers
   Chemicals which influence blood flow to muscle or affect ATP
7. Modulation of glial cell production of cytokines and its influence upon opiates
8. Electrical brain stimulation
   Transcranial magnetic stimulation
   Direct current stimulation
   Vagal nerve stimulation

underlying abnormality. (The only known exception to this is that it appears as though the opioidergic systems are appropriately hyperactive in FM patients, which may explain why opioidergic drugs show little efficacy in this and related conditions). Also, glial cell activity cannot be measured by any blood testing, as it occurs entirely within the blood-brain barrier. There is evidence that modulation of glial cells and its ability to produce cytokines make one resistant to opiates represents an important area for future investigation. There have been several studies suggesting that therapies that stimulate specific brain or nervous system structures can improve pain and other symptoms in FM. These include Transcranial Magnetic Stimulation (TMS), and Direct Current Stimulation (DCS), two therapies that stimulate underlying brain regions using magnetic influences or direct current. These therapies appear to be well tolerated in early studies, although there is a theoretical risk of inducing seizures. Other similar therapies such as Vagal Nerve Stimulation (VNS) are also under study in FM.

These approaches are summarized in Table 25.1. All of these preparations potentially are capable of decreasing pain and diminishing pain perception. Over the next 20–30 years, gene manipulation and control over apoptosis (programmed cell death) will challenge ethicists and scientists as we become capable of fundamentally manipulating our genes, cells, and progeny—thus, perhaps, greatly reducing the properties and production of pain.

Fibromyalgia patients should not give up hope. We've come so far in the last decade. Now, new exciting challenges are just beginning!

FOR FURTHER READING

Bazzichi L, Sernissi F, Consensi A, *et al.* Fibromyalgia: A critical digest of the recent literature. *Clin Exp Rheumatol* 2011; *29* (Supp 69), S1–S11.

Clauw DJ. Pharmacotherapy for patients with fibromyalgia. *J Clin Psychiatry* 2008; *69* (supp 2); 25–29.

Hsu MC, Clauw DJ. A different type of procedure for a different type of pain. *Arthritis Rheum* 2006; *54*: 3725–3727.

Recia JM. New and emerging therapeutic agents for the treatment of fibromyalgia: an update, *J Pain Research* 2010; *3*: 89–103.

Appendix 1: Resource Information

The organizations listed below can be readily accessed via their websites through any search engine:

Non-profit organizations that fund fibromyalgia research and training or promote patient advocacy and education and have a budget of over $1 million a year. Some of those listed also publish peer-review journals

Arthritis Foundation, 1330 W Peachtree St #100, Atlanta, GA 30309, 800-283-7800. There are 56 U.S. chapters which provide research monies, publish literature, and offer patient support for arthritis and related conditions such as lupus. Website: www.arthritis.org

American College of Rheumatology (ACR), 2200 Lake Blvd NE, Atlanta, GA 30319, 404-633-3777. This is the professional organization to which nearly all U.S. and many international rheumatologists belong. Website: www.rheumatology.org or call toll-free 800- 346-4753.

National Institute of Arthritis and Musculoskeletal and Skin Diseases (NIAMS), Bldg. 31, Room 4C02, 31 Center Drive MSC 2350, Bethesda, MD 20892. Part of the National Institutes of Health, NIAMS funds $90 million dollars in fibromyalgia research each year at the Bethesda campus and elsewhere in the country. 301-496-8190. Website: www.niams.nih.gov

Fibromyalgia Network, P.O. Box 31750, Tucson, AZ 85751-1750, 520-290-5508 or 800-853-2929, supports research through the American Fibromyalgia Syndrome Association. Website: www.fmnetnews.com/

American Pain Society 4700 W. Lake Ave., Glenview, IL 60025, 847-375-4715. Fax: 877-734-8758, www.ampainsoc.org is a multidisciplinary organization of professional pain specialists. It publishes the *Journal of Pain*.

National Fibromyalgia and Chronic Pain Association is the largest membership organization for fibromyalgia patients in the United States. 31 Federal Ave, Logan Utah, 84521. www.fmcpaware.org, 1-800-200-3727.

Who are the editors of rheumatology textbooks that devote considerable space to fibromyalgia and related topics?

Wallace DJ, Clauw DJ, eds. *Fibromyalgia and Other Central Pain Syndromes* (Lippincott Williams & Wilkins, 2005)

Hochberg MC, Silman AJ, Smolen JS, Weinblatt, ME, Weisman MH, eds. *Rheumatology–2 Volume Set, 5th Edition* (Elsevier 2010).

Harris ED Jr, Budd RC, Firestein G, *et al. Kelley's Textbook of Rheumatology* (WB Saunders, 2004)

Koopman WJ, Moreland LW. *Arthritis and Allied Conditions: A Textbook of Rheumatology, 15th Edition* (Lippincott Williams & Wilkins, 2004).

Isenberg D, Maddison PJ, Woo P, Glass D, Breedvald F, *Oxford Textbook of Rheumatology, 3rd Edition* (Oxford University Press, 2004)

Clauw DJ, Wallace DJ, *Fibromyalgia: The Essential Clinician's Guide*. (Oxford American Rheumatology Library, 2009)

Choy E, *Fibromyalgia* (Oxford University Press, 2009).

Which other medical journals publish a substantial number of peer-reviewed articles relating to fibromyalgia?

Annals of the Rheumatic Diseases

Journal of Musculoskeletal Pain

Journal of Rheumatology

Rheumatology

Journal of Pain

Arthritis and Rheumatism

Arthritis Care and Research

Appendix 2: Glossary

acetylcholine a neurotransmitter of the autonomic nervous system (see below) that induces dilation of blood vessels and slows down the gastrointestinal and urinary tracts.

affective spectrum disorder a term used to consider irritable bowel, tension headache, irritable bladder, premenstrual tension, and fibromyalgia as being primarily of behavioral and secondarily of physiologic causation.

afferent nerves nerves going from the periphery (e.g., skin, muscle) toward the spine.

alexithymia long-standing personality disorder with generalized and localized complaints in individuals who cannot express underlying psychological conflicts.

allodynia what happens when something that should not hurt causes pain. Fibromyalgia is chronic, widespread allodynia.

alpha/delta sleep wave abnormality delta waves make up most of slow wave, or nondream, sleep. Alpha waves interrupting delta waves can produce movement or awakening, leading to unrefreshing sleep.

American College of Rheumatology (ACR) a professional association of 5,000 American rheumatologists and 2,000 allied health professionals (the Association of Rheumatology Health Professionals).

Arthritis Foundation a nonprofit national organization that provides patient support and funds research on musculoskeletal disorders.

autonomic nervous system (ANS) part of the peripheral nervous system and divided into sympathetic and parasympathetic components. Regulates stress responses, sweat, urine, and bowel reflexes and determines if a blood vessel constricts or dilates, thereby affecting pulse and blood pressure.

B cell a white blood cell that makes antibodies.

benzodiazepine an anxiolytic group of drugs, including diazepam (Valium) and clonazepam (Klonopin), that relaxes muscles, among other actions, by blocking GABA (see below).

biofeedback   a training technique enabling an individual to gain some voluntary control over autonomic body functions.

body dysmorphic disorder   a condition of individuals engrossed with themselves who express excessive concern or fear over having a defect in appearance.

bradykinins   chemicals that mediate inflammation and dilate blood vessels.

bruxism   persistently grinding one's teeth.

bursa   a sac of synovial fluid between tendons, muscles, and bones that promotes easier movement.

candida hypersensitivity syndrome   a controversial condition based on theories that a toxin released by yeast is responsible for irritable bowel, fatigue, and a feeling of illness. Candida is a type of yeast, or fungus.

carpal tunnel syndrome   compression of the median nerve as it traverses the palmar side of the wrist, producing shooting nerve pains in the first to fourth fingers.

cartilage   tissue material that covers bone.

causalgia   sustained burning pain, allodynia, and overreaction to stimuli associated with autonomic nervous system dysfunction. Reflex sympathetic dystrophy is chronic, widespread causalgia.

Centers for Disease Control (CDC)   an agency of the federal government based in Atlanta that monitors, defines, and sets standards for managing epidemics, infections, new diseases, and certain types of blood tests.

Central sensitization syndrome   a group of local and systemic syndromes characterized by amplification of sensory afferent input resulting in pain.

chiropractic   a therapy involving manipulation of spine and joints to influence the body's nervous system and natural defense mechanisms.

chronic fatigue immune dysfunction syndrome (CFIDS)   a controversial term for chronic fatigue syndrome implying a prominent role for immune abnormalities.

chronic fatigue syndrome (CFS)   unexplained fatigue lasting for more than six months associated with musculoskeletal and systemic symptoms. Most of these patients fulfill the criteria for fibromyalgia.

cognitive behavioral therapy   the use of biofeedback-related techniques to improve speech and memory.

cognitive dysfunction   difficulty focusing, remembering names or dates, performing numerical calculations, or articulating clearly.

collagen   structural protein found in bone, cartilage, and skin.

conversion reaction   a form of hysteria whereby an emotion is transformed into a physical manifestation (e.g., a person with normal vision claiming that "I can't see").

corticosteroid   any anti-inflammatory hormone made by the adrenal gland's cortex, or center.

corticotropin-releasing hormone (CRH) a chemical made in the hypothalamus of the brain that ultimately leads to the release of steroids by the adrenal gland.

cortisone a synthetic corticosteroid.

costochondritis irritation of the tethering tissues connecting the sternum (breastbone) to the ribs, producing chest pains; also called Tietze's syndrome.

cytokines proteins that act as messenger chemicals of the immune system.

delta sleep a type of electrical wave found on a tracing of brain waves during nondream sleep.

depression helplessness and hopelessness leading to feelings of worthlessness, loss of appetite, alterations in sleep patterns, loss of self-esteem, inability to concentrate, complaints of fatigue, and loss of energy.

disability a limitation of function that compromises the ability to perform an activity within a range considered normal.

dorsal horn nerves inside the back of the spinal cord. These run from the brain to the waist area.

dorsal root ganglion nerve cell bodies in the peripheral nervous system that receive nociceptive inputs and transmit them to the spinal cord.

dynorphin an opiate that suppresses acute pain but perpetuates chronic pain.

dysautonomia abnormal function of the autonomic nervous system.

dysmenorrhea painful periods.

edema swelling of tissues, usually due to inflammation or fluid retention.

efferent nerves nerves that go from the spinal cord to its periphery.

electroencephalogram (EEG) a mapping of electrical activity within the brain.

electromyogram (EMG) a map of electrical activity within muscles. Usually combined with a *nerve conduction velocity* study, which assesses nerve damage or injury.

endorphin chemical substance in the brain that acts as an opiate. Relieves pain by raising the body's pain threshold.

enkephalin similar to endorphin (see above).

eosinophilia myalgic syndrome (EMS) a scleroderma-like thickening of fascia (see below) associated with high levels of circulating eosinophils caused by a contaminant of L-tryptophan. Many patients with EMS develop fibromyalgia.

epidemiology study of relationships between various factors that determine who gets a disorder and how many people have it.

epinephrine or adrenalin, a "nerve hormone" produced in the adrenal gland that acts as a neurotransmitter and stimulates the sympathetic nervous system.

Epstein-Barr virus (EBV) a herpesvirus producing a mononucleosis-like illness that can lead to chronic fatigue syndrome.

ergonomics   a discipline that studies the relationship between human factors, the design and operation of machines, behavior, and the physical environment.

erythrocyte sedimentation rate (ESR)   see sedimentation rate.

excitatory amino acids   such as glutamate and aspartate function as neurotransmitting chemicals in chronic pain. When they are blocked, fibromyalgia pain is relieved.

fascia   a layer of tissue between skin and muscle.

female urethral syndrome   or irritable bladder; persistent urge to void without evidence of infection, obstruction, stricture, or inflammation.

fever a   temperature above 99.6⁰F.

fibromyalgia   chronic, widespread, amplified pain associated with fatigue, sleep disorder, tender points, and systemic symptoms.

fibrositis   an outdated term for fibromyalgia (see above); discarded since it implies inflammation, which is usually not present.

flare   reappearance of symptoms; another word for exacerbation.

gamma-aminobutyric acid (GABA)   an inhibitory neurotransmitter.

gate theory   blocking or regulating transmission of pain impulses in the dorsal horn of the spinal column.

gene   consisting of DNA, it is the basic unit of inherited information in our cells.

Gulf War syndrome   a fibromyalgia-like disorder among Gulf War (1991) veterans probably caused by taking a combination of medicines meant to protect them from chemical warfare.

handicap   a job limitation; something that prevents one from doing something.

homeopathy   a discipline based on the idea that symptoms can be eliminated by taking infinitesimal amounts of substances that, in large amounts, would produce the same symptoms.

hormones   chemical messengers made by the body, including thyroid, steroids, insulin, estrogen, progesterone, and testosterone.

hyperalgesia   exaggerated response to a painful stimulus.

hypermobility   laxity of ligaments allowing one to assume positions or undertake movements difficult for a normal person to do.

hyperpathia   delayed or persistent pain from noxious stimuli.

hypochondriasis   excessive preoccupation with the fear of having a serious disease based on misinterpretation of one or more bodily symptoms or signs.

hypoglycemia   low blood sugar level.

hypothalamic-pituitary-adrenal (HPA) axis   the system by which a releasing hormone secreted by the hypothalamus induces the pituitary gland to secrete stimulating hormone, which, in turn, induces the adrenal glands to release steroid-related hormones.

hypothalamus a region of the brain that produces chemicals which result in the release of hormones.

hypoxia insufficient oxygen reaching a tissue, organ, or region of the body.

hysteria see conversion reaction.

impairment an anatomic, physiologic, or psychological loss that leads to disability.

incidence the rate at which a population develops a disorder.

Interferon a protein with antiviral activity and has immune regulatory properties that can produce cognitive impairment and aching.

interleukin protein substances that are intercellular mediators of inflammation and the immune response.

interstitial cystitis a chronic inflammatory condition of the bladder.

irritable bladder see female urethral syndrome.

irritable bowel syndrome symptoms of abdominal distention, bloating, mucus-containing stools, and irregular bowel habits without an obvious cause.

leaky gut syndrome a controversial entity based on the belief that an overload of poisons overwhelms the liver's ability to detoxify, making the intestinal lining more permeable.

ligament a tether attaching bone to bone, giving them stability.

limbic system a collection of brain structures that influences endocrine and autonomic systems and affects motivational and mood states.

livedo reticularis a lace-like pattern of small veins and capillaries visible on the skin.

lupus (also systemic lupus erythematosus [SLE]) an autoimmune multisystemic disease caused by abnormal immune regulation resulting in tissue damage.

Lyme disease caused when a deer-borne tick infects people with a bacterium; it is frequently associated with fibromyalgia and fatigue syndromes.

lymphadenopathy swollen, palpable lymph nodes.

lymphocyte a type of white blood cell that fights infection and mediates the immune response.

magnetic resonance imaging (MRI) a picture of a body region derived from using magnets; involves no radiation.

melatonin a substance made by the pineal gland of the brain that promotes sleep.

migraine a vascular headache.

mitral valve prolapse a floppy heart valve that can produce palpitations.

multiple chemical sensitivity syndrome a controversial condition suggesting that chemicals in the environment produce symptoms and signs at levels not thought to be harmful.

myalgia pain in the muscles.

myelinated fibers a fat-protein sheath surrounding nerve fibers.

myoclonus   twitching of a muscle or a group of muscles.

myofascial pain   discomfort in the muscles and fascia.

myofascial pain syndrome   fibromyalgia-like pain limited to one region of the body; also known as regional myofascial pain.

National Institutes of Health (NIH)   a federal government organization that funds medical research.

neurally mediated hypotension   low blood pressure due to autonomic dysfunction.

neurokinins   substances made by nerves having physiologic effects.

neuropathic   pathology produced by compression, damage, or destruction of a nerve.

neuropeptides   consist of short chemical sequences common to amino acids (a building block of protein) that have effects on one's perception of pain and can act as neurotransmitters.

neuroplasticity   central brain sensitization that, if prolonged, produces phantom limb pain.

neurotransmitters   chemical substances that transmit messages through nerves.

nerve conduction velocity (NCV)   measures the rate of nerve transmission and is usually part of an electromyogram (see above).

NMDA (N-methyl-D-aspartate) receptor   a neurotransmitter sensor or receptor different from opiates that interacts with excitatory amino acids (see above).

nociceptor   a nerve that receives and transmits painful stimuli. Nociception is the process that transmits stimuli from the periphery (skin, muscles, tissues) to the central nervous system.

nonrestorative sleep   waking up feeling unrefreshed.

nonsteroidal anti-inflammatory   drugs (NSAIDs) agents such as aspirin, ibuprofen, or naproxen that fight inflammation by blocking the actions of prostaglandin.

norepinephrine   a "nerve hormone" produced in the adrenal gland that acts as a neurotransmitter and stimulates the autonomic nervous system.

obsessive-compulsive disorder (OCD)   persistent ideas or impulses; can include performing repetitive acts or having perfectionistic tendencies.

occupational therapy   uses ergonomics in designing tasks to fit the capabilities of the human body.

opiates   narcotics.

osteopath   a physician who is trained in performing specialized physical manipulative modalities.

overuse syndrome   pain in muscles, ligaments, tendons, or joints from excessive activity in an area of the body.

pain   an unpleasant sensation or emotional experience.

palindromic rheumatism   intermittent swelling or inflammation of joints.

palmar erythema   redness of the hands due to an autonomic reaction.

parasympathetic nervous system a   division of the autonomic nervous system that blocks acetylcholine.

paresthesia a   sensation of numbness, tingling, burning, or prickling anywhere in the body.

peripheral nervous system   nerves to and from the spinal cord that transmit sensation and motor reflexes.

physiatrist   a practitioner of physical medicine (see below).

physical medicine   a medical specialty concerned with the principles of musculoskeletal, cardiovascular, and neurologic rehabilitation.

physical therapist   allied health professional that assists patients with physical conditioning.

pituitary   a gland in the brain that assists in the production of hormones.

pleuritis   inflammation or irritation of the lining of the lung.

polymyalgia rheumatica   an autoimmune disease of the joints and muscles seen in older patients with high sedimentation rates who have aching in their shoulders, upper arms, hips, and upper legs.

polymyositis   an autoimmune, inflammatory disorder of muscles.

positron emission tomography (PET)   an imaging technique that measures the flow of a substance to tissues

prednisone; prednisolone   synthetic steroids.

premenstrual syndrome (PMS)   the release of chemicals prior to menstruation, causing fluid retention, alterations in mood and behavior, and sometimes painful periods.

prevalence   the number of people who have a condition or disorder per unit of population.

primary fibromyalgia syndrome   fibromyalgia of unknown cause.

prolactin a   hormone that stimulates the secretion of breast milk.

prostaglandins   physiologically active substances present in many tissues.

protein a collection   of amino acids. Antibodies are proteins.

psychogenic rheumatism   complaints of joint pain for purposes of secondary gain.

psychosomatic   when parts of the brain or mind influence functions of the body.

rapid eye movement (REM) sleep   the part of sleep in which we may dream.

Raynaud's disease   Isolated Raynaud's phenomenon (see below); not part of any other disease.

Raynaud's phenomenon   discoloration of the hands or feet (which turn blue, white, or red), especially with stress or cold temperatures; a feature of many autoimmune diseases.

reactive hyperemia   increased blood flow to an area following prior interruption or compromise of circulation.

referred pain   perceived as coming from an area different from its actual origin.

reflex sympathetic dystrophy (RSD) a   type of fibromyalgia associated with sustained burning pain and swelling, also called complex regional pain syndrome, Type 1.

reflexology   a form of alternative medicine based on the theory that specific areas of the ears, hands, and feet correspond to organs, glands, and nerves.

regional myofascial syndrome   fibromyalgia pain limited to one region of the body; also known as *myofascial pain syndrome.*

repetitive strain syndrome   when repetitive motions in a work environment produce strain or stress on an area of the body, as in carpal tunnel syndrome from excessive typing.

restless legs syndrome   a form of periodic limb movement syndrome, in which legs suddenly shoot out, lift, jerk, or go into spasm. If this occurs during sleep, it is called sleep myoclonus.

seasonal affective disorder   when light deprivation during winter months produces depression and fatigue.

sedimentation rate   test that measures the rate of fall of red blood cells in a column of blood; high rates indicate inflammation or infection.

selective serotonin reuptake inhibitor (SSRI)   a class of drugs that treat depression and pain by boosting serotonin levels.

serotonin   a chemical that aids sleep, reduces pain, and influences mood and appetite. Derived from tryptophan and stored in blood platelets.

Sicca syndrome   dry eyes. Can be due to decreased sympathetic nervous system activity, medication or Sjogren's syndrome (see below).

sick building syndrome   allergy and fibromyalgia-like symptoms complained of by more than one person with extreme sensitivity to environmental components in the same home or workplace.

single photon emission computed tomography (SPECT)   an imaging study that measures flow of oxygen to the brain

Sjogren's syndrome   dry eyes, dry mouth, and arthritis observed in many autoimmune disorders or by itself (primary Sjogren's).

sleep myoclonus   restless legs syndrome (see above) that occurs during sleep.

slow wave sleep a   phase of sleep not associated with dreaming but with alpha waves on an electroencephalogram (see above).

soft tissue rheumatism   musculoskeletal complaints relating to tendons, muscles, bursae, ligaments, and fascial tissues. Includes fibromyalgia.

somatization   conversion of anxiety and other psychological states into physical symptoms.

somatomedin C   a form of growth hormone.

somatotropin   growth hormone.

spinoreticular tract   a trail of nerves that conducts impulses to the brain that regulate the autonomic nervous system from the periphery.

spinothalamic tract   a trail of nerves that conveys impulses to the brain associated with touch, pain, and temperature.

steroids   shortened term for corticosteroids, which are anti-inflammatory hormones produced by the adrenal gland's cortex or synthetically.

substance P   a neurotransmitter chemical that increases pain perception.

sympathetic nervous system (SNS)   a branch of the autonomic nervous system that regulates the release of norepinephrine (see above).

syndrome   a constellation of associated symptoms, signs, and laboratory findings.

synovitis   inflammation of the tissues lining a joint.

synovium   tissue that lines the joint.

taut band   a tight, rubber-band-like knot in the muscles.

T cell   a lymphocyte responsible for immunologic memory.

temporomandibular joint   **(TMJ) dysfunction syndrome** pain in the jaw joint associated with localized myofascial discomfort.

tender point   an area of tenderness in the muscles, tendons, bony prominences, or fat pads.

tendon   structure that attaches muscle to bone.

thalamus   an oval mass of gray matter in the brain that receives signals from nerve tracts in the spinal cord.

Tietze's syndrome   another term for costochondritis (see above).

tinnitus   ringing in the ears.

titer   amount of a substance.

tricyclic   a family of antidepressant drugs such as Elavil that relieve depression, promote restful sleep, relax muscles, and raise the pain threshold.

Trigger point   an area of muscle that, when touched, triggers a reaction of discomfort

tryptophan   an amino acid that can be broken down to serotonin.

vaginismus   tightness of the vaginal muscles, which prevents or limits penetration during sexual intercourse.

vertigo   malfunction of the vestibular (balance center) of the ear, producing a sensation that everything around you is in motion.

visceral hyperalgesia   pain amplification mediated by the parasympathetic nervous system thought to cause irritable bowel and ulcer-like symptoms.

vocational rehabilitation   training someone for an occupation, which takes into account the person's educational background and physical skills, as well as his or her handicaps or impairnents.

vulvodynia   pain in the female genital area when infection, cancer, stricture, or inflammation has been ruled out.

Index

In this index "FM" refers to fibromyalgia; "*f*" after the page number indicates a figure; "*t*" indicates a table.